CENTRAL NERVOUS SYSTEM LEUKEMIA

DEVELOPMENTS IN ONCOLOGY

F.J. Cleton and J.W.I.M. Simons, eds., Genetic Origins of Tumour Cells
ISBN 90-247-2272-1
J. Aisner and P. Chang, eds., Cancer Treatment Research
ISBN 90-247-2358-2
B.W. Ongerboer de Visser, D.A. Bosch and W.M.H. van Woerkom-Eykenboom, eds.,
Neuro-oncology: Clinical and Experimental Aspects
ISBN 90-247-2421-X
K. Hellmann, P. Hilgard and S. Eccles, eds., Metastasis: Clinical and Experimental Aspects
ISBN 90-247-2424-4
H.F. Seigler, ed., Clinical Management of Melanoma
ISBN 90-247-2584-4
P. Correa and W. Haenszel, eds., Epidemiology of Cancer of the Digestive Tract
ISBN 90-247-2601-8
L.A. Liotta and I.R. Hart, eds., Tumour Invasion and Metastasis
ISBN 90-247-2611-5
J. Bánóczy, ed., Oral Leukoplakia
ISBN 90-247-2655-7
C. Tijssen, M. Halprin and L. Endtz, eds., Familial Brain Tumours
ISBN 90-247-2691-3
F.M. Muggia, C.W. Young and S.K. Carter, eds., Anthracycline Antibiotics in Cancer
ISBN 90-247-2711-1
B.W. Hancock, ed., Assessment of Tumour Response
ISBN 90-247-2712-X
D.E. Peterson, ed., Oral Complications of Cancer Chemotherapy
ISBN 0-89838-563-6

CENTRAL NERVOUS SYSTEM LEUKEMIA

Prevention and Treatment

edited by

RENATO MASTRANGELO, MD
Clinica Pediatrica, Università Cattolica, Roma, Italy

DAVID G. POPLACK, MD
Pediatric Oncology Branch,
National Cancer Institute
Bethesda, MD 20205
USA

RICCARDO RICCARDI, MD
Clinica Pediatrica, Università Cattolica, Roma, Italy

1983 **MARTINUS NIJHOFF PUBLISHERS**
a member of the KLUWER ACADEMIC PUBLISHERS GROUP
BOSTON / THE HAGUE / DORDRECHT / LANCASTER

Distributors

for the United States and Canada: Kluwer Boston, Inc., 190 Old Derby Street, Hingham, MA 02043, USA
for all other countries: Kluwer Academic Publishers Group, Distribution Center,P.O.Box 322, 3300 AH Dordrecht, The Netherlands

Library of Congress Cataloging in Publication Data   CIP

Main entry under title:

Central nervous system leukemia.

   (Developments in oncology ; v. 13)
   Includes index.
   1. Lymphoblastic leukemia in children--Treatment.
2. Central nervous system--Cancer--Prevention.
I. Mastrangelo, Renato. II. Poplack, David G.
III. Riccardi, Riccardo, 1897-   . IV. Series.
[DNLM: 1. Central nervous system diseases--Prevention
and control. 2. Central nervous system diseases--
Therapy. 3. Leukemia, Lymphoblastic--Prevention and
 control. 4. Leukemia, Lymphoblastic--Therapy. W1
 DE998N v. 13 / WH 250 C397]
 RJ416.L4C46 1983   616.89'99419   83-2425

ISBN-13: 978-94-009-6710-6   e-ISBN-13: 978-94-009-6708-3
DOI: 10.1007/978-94-009-6708-3

Copyright

Table of Contents

Preface VII

List of Contributors IX

1. The Pathology of Central Nervous System Leukemia 1
   R.A. PRICE

2. Radiation Therapy Methods for Central Nervous System 'Prophylaxis' in the Management of Childhood Leukemias 11
   G.J. D'ANGIO

3. Central Nervous System Prophylaxis for Therapy of Acute Lymphocytic Leukemia 17
   A.M. MAUER, J. OCHS, W.P. BOWMAN, L. CH'IEN, W. EVANS, R. RAGLAND, R. BERG, L. PARVEY, TH. CORBURN and J.V. SIMONE

4. Reduction in Central Nervous System Leukemia with a Pharmacokinetically derived Intrathecal-Methotrexate Dosage Regimen 27
   W.A. BLEYER, C. LEVEL, H.N. SATHER, D.J. NIEBRUGGE, P.F. COCCIA, S. SIEGEL, PH.S. LITTMAN, S.L. LEIKIN, D.R. MILLER, R.L. CHARD, Jr. and G. DENMAN HAMMOND

5. Central Nervous System Prophylaxis with Intermittent Intrathecal Methotrexate and Fractional Radiation in Childhood Acute Lymphoblastic Leukemia 39
   Y. RAVINDRANATH, K. BHAMBHANI, JOHN K. KELLY, G. SCHULTZ, I. WARRIER, B. CONSIDINE, J.M. LUSHER and W.W. ZUELZER

6. Intermittent Intrathecal Methotrexate and Fractional Radiation plus Chemotherapy in Childhood Lymphoblastic Leukemia 49
   R. MASTRANGELO, R. RICCARDI, R. MALANDRINO and A. ROMANINI

7.   Prophylaxis of Central Nervous System Leukaemia: British Experience, 1970–80   53
     R.M. HARDISTY

8.   The Norwegian Methotrexate Study in Childhood Acute Lymphocytic Leukemia   63
     P.J. MOE, M. SEIP, P.H. FINNE and S. KOLMANNSKOG

9.   Therapy Related Central Nervous System Diseases in Children with Acute Lymphocytic Leukemia   71
     R.A. PRICE

10. Neurotoxic Complications of CNS Prophylaxis in Childhood Leukaemia   83
     M.G. MOTT

11. Evaluation of Adverse Sequelae of Central Nervous System Prophylaxis in Acute Lymphoblastic Leukemia   95
     D.G. POPLACK

12. Adverse Sequelae of Central Nervous System Prophylaxis in Acute Lymphoblastic Leukemia   105
     G. PAOLUCCI and P. ROSITO

13. Treatment of Overt CNS Leukaemia   113
     M.L.N. WILLOUGHBY

14. Radiation Therapy Methods for the Treatment of Central Nervous System Leukemia   123
     A. OAKHILL and G.J. D'ANGIO

15. Treatment of Meningeal Leukemia: Investigation of New Approaches with Conventional Agents   131
     R. RICCARDI and D.G. POPLACK

Subject Index   137

Preface

In the past 10 to 15 years there has been dramatic improvement in the survival of children with acute lymphoblastic leukemia. At the present time, over 50% of children with this disease will be alive and free of their disease at least 5 years from the time of their initial diagnosis. Although a number of factors have contributed to this improvement, perhaps none has been as important as the institution of central nervous system preventive therapy (CNS prophylaxis). However, despite the efficacy of CNS prophylaxis, the prevention and treatment of central nervous system leukemia continues to pose a formidable clinical challenge to the pediatric oncologist. Although successful in most cases, CNS preventive therapy remains ineffective for a small but significant subset of patients at high risk for developing CNS disease. Moreover, it has become increasingly evident that some methods of CNS preventive therapy are associated with long-term, adverse CNS sequelae. Thus, considerable controversy exists regarding the optimal method of CNS prophylaxis.

Treatment of the patient who develops overt meningeal leukemia has not been as successful and continues to pose a major clinical challenge. Despite the ability of intrathecal chemotherapy and/or radiation therapy to induce CNS remission, most patients suffer subsequent relapse and ultimate survival is usually significantly compromised. It is evident that newer approaches to treatment for this patient group must be identified before major improvement for this patient group is likely to occur.

In late 1981, a group of leading clinical investigators was brought together in a unique workshop in an attempt to examine the topic of the prevention and treatment of central nervous system leukemia. An important goal of the workshop was to prepare a book which would summarize and review controversial areas in this field. We are hopeful that the papers selected for inclusion in this book will provide the type of perspective that will lead to new insights and hopefully to therapeutic improvement in the future.

January, 1983   THE EDITORS

List of Contributors

W.A. BLEYER, Associate Professor of Pediatrics, University of Washington, Department of Haematology – Oncology, Children's Hospital Orthopedic Medical Center, Seattle WA 98105, USA
(co-authors: C. Level, H.N. Sather, D.J. Niebrugge, P.F. Coccia, S. Siegel, Ph.S. Littman, S.L. Leikin, D.R. Miller, R.L. Chard Jr., G.D. Hammond)

G.J. D'ANGIO, Director, Children's Cancer Research Center, Children's Hospital of Philadelphia, Civic Center Boulevard, Philadelphia PA 19104, USA

R.M. HARDISTY, Department of Haematology, Institute of Child Health and Hospital for Sick Children, Great Ormond Street, London WC1N 3JH, Great Britain

R. MASTRANGELO, Associate Professor, Department of Pediatrics, Catholic University of Rome, 00168 Rome, Italy
(co-authors: R. Riccardi, R. Malandrino; A. Romanini, Instituto di Radiologia, Catholic University of Rome)

A.V. MAUER, Director, St. Jude Children's Research Hospital, 332 North Lauderdale, Memphis, TN 38101, USA
(co-authors: J. Ochs, W.P. Bowman, L. Ch'ien, W. Evans, R. Ragland, R. Berg, L. Parvey, Th. Coburn, J.V. Simone)

P.J. MOE, Professor, Department of Pediatrics Regionsykehuset, University of Trondheim, Trondheim, Norway
(co-authors: M. Seip, Department of Pediatrics, Rikshospitalet, University of Oslo; P.H. Finne, Department of Pediatrics, Haukeland Sykehus, University of Bergen; S. Kolmannskog, Department of Pediatrics, University of Tromsø, Norway)

M.G. MOTT, Senior Lecturer in Child Health, University of Bristol, Bristol BS8 1TD, Great Britain

G. PAOLUCCI, Director, Department of Pediatrics, University of Bologna, Bologna, Italy
(co-author: P. Rosito)

D.G. POPLACK, Head, Leukemia Biology Section, Pediatric Oncology Branch, National Cancer Institute, Bethesda MD 20205, USA

ROBERT A. PRICE, Associate Professor of Pathology, University of Pittsburgh,

School of Medicine and Neuropathologist, Children's Hospital of Pittsburgh, Pittsburgh, PA 15213, USA

Y. RAVINDRANATH, Haematology – Oncology Division, Children's Hospital of Michigan, 3901 Beaubien Boulevard, Detroit, MI 48201, USA
(co-authors: K. Bhambhani, J.K. Kelly, G. Schultz, I. Warrier, B. Considine, J.M. Lusher, W.W. Zuelzer)

R. RICCARDI, Assistant Professor of Pediatrics, Catholic University of Rome, 00168 Rome, Italy

M.L.N. WILLOUGHBY, Consultant Haematologist, Royal Hospital for Sick Children, Glasgow, Great Britain

A. OAKHILL, Consultant Pediatric Haematologist – Oncologist, Bristol Royal Children's Hospital, Bristol, Great Britain

1. The Pathology of Central Nervous System Leukemia

R.A. PRICE

Summary

Invasion of the leptomeninges by leukemic cells is an early and common complication in children who develop acute lymphocytic leukemia. If not adequately treated this disease progresses and produces characteristic anatomical sequelae and predictable clinical manifestations. This paper has reviewed these problems by examining a) the anatomy of the leptomeninges as it pertains to CNS leukemia, b) the sequence of events occurring during the histopathogenesis of meningeal leukemia, and c) the histological sequelae and their resultant clinical manifestations.

Introduction

Central nervous system leukemia is defined as leukemic invasion of the leptomeninges, with or without infiltration of adjacent neural tissue (1). Numerous studies indicate that leukemic cells follow a predictable anatomical course during invasion of the central nervous system (CNS) with predictable anatomical lesions and resultant clinical manifestations. Sufficient data exist to assume that leukemic cells have invaded the leptomeninges by the time of initial hematological diagnosis of this disorder or shortly thereafter (2–7).

This presentation will review a) the structure of the leptomeninges as it pertains to CNS leukemia, b) the sequence of histological events and the pathogenesis of CNS leukemia, and c) the sequelae of these histopathological lesions in CNS tissue and the resultant clinical manifestations (or complications) attributable to them.

The leptomeninges

Central nervous system leukemia is a disease of the leptomeninges. The morphological lesions and the clinical sequelae of arachnoid leukemia are related to the structural features of the leptomeninges. The presence of the subarachnoid

R. Mastrangelo, D.G. Poplack, R. Riccardi (eds), Central Nervous System Leukemia. ISBN 978-94-009-6710-6.
© *1983 Martinus Nijhoff Publishers, Boston.*

space makes possible the clinical, cytological diagnosis of meningeal leukemia in both symptomatic and asymptomatic patients.

The leptomeninges are composed of arachnoid and pia mater. The arachnoid consists of two parts: 1) a surface membrane and connective tissue trabeculae through which vessels and nerves pass, and 2) mesothelial lined channels through which the cerebrospinal fluid (CSF) flows. The arachnoid membrane has two distinct topographical divisions: a) a superficial portion covering the surfaces of the brain, and b) a deep portion, which surrounds vessels penetrating or emerging from gray and white matter of the brain and forming the true perivascular, or Virchow-Robin, space. The majority of CSF channels, including large cisterns, are located in the superficial portion of the arachnoid. These channels cannot be consistently identified in the deep portions. This anatomical distinction of two divisions may be of considerable importance in the treatment of CNS leukemia, since these are the principal channels for the intrathecal passage of drugs used in the treatment of meningeal leukemia.

CNS tissue is tightly encased by the pial-glial membrane which separates the arachnoid from neural tissue. This membrane extends deeply into the parenchyma and merges with the adventitia of the precapillary arteriole and postcapillary venule. With few exceptions (e.g. in the circumventricular organs) capillaries in the brain are not surrounded by leptomeninges. It is in the capillaries of the CNS vasculature that the blood-brain-barrier (BBB) is located. The BBB possesses unique physiological characteristics and is composed of capillary endothelium, a basement membrane, and glial processes from adjacent astrocytes. The BBB should not be confused with the blood-CSF-barrier, located in the choroid plexus, which produces most of the CSF.

Histopathology and pathogenesis

The consistent finding of leukemic cells in the walls of leptomeningeal vessels led Dr. Fried in 1926 to postulate that cells circulating in the blood pass through vessel walls and invade the surrounding tissues of the brain (5). Leukemic cells in the walls of veins in the superficial leptomeninges are indeed the first histologic evidence of CNS leukemia (Figure 1). Certain clinical features and related autopsy observations indicate that invasion of the superficial leptomeninges is present at the time of diagnosis of leukemia, or occurs shortly thereafter. During these early stages of infiltration, only the superficial portions of the leptomeninges are affected. Deeper arachnoid along the blood vessels within gray and white matter is free of malignant cells. The arachnoid trabeculae are intact and the CSF itself remains free of leukemic cells.

This leukemic infiltration eventually leads to destruction of the trabeculae with the release of cells into the CSF so that the cytological diagnosis of meningeal leukemia is possible. As early as 1935 Schwab and Weiss (3) concluded that

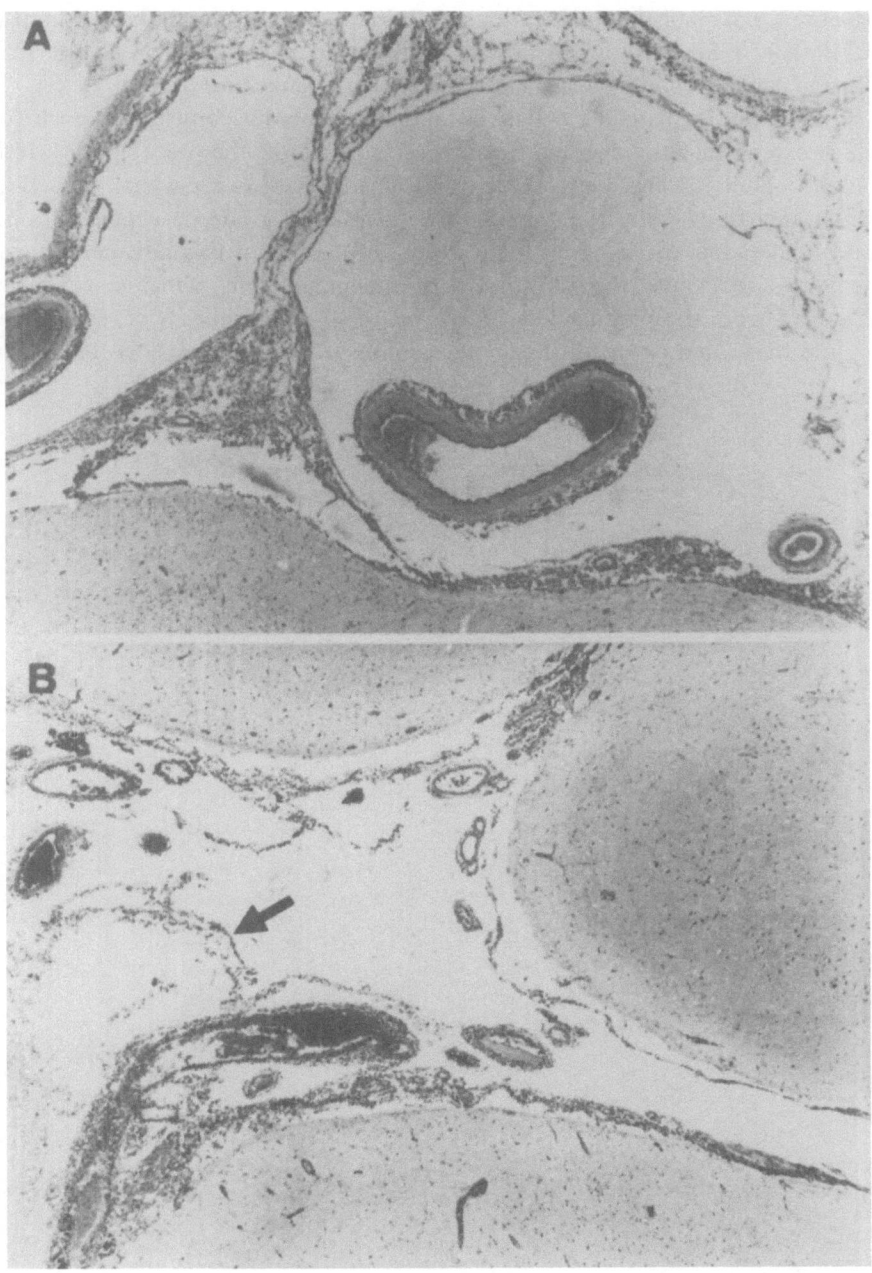

Figure 1. A. Minimal leukemic infiltration of arachnoid trabeculae with no leukemic cells in CSF channels. A cellular infiltrate surrounds a normal artery. Verhoeff's elastic tissue stain. × 32. B. Distortion of trabeculae by leukemic cells (arrow) and contamination of CSF channels. HE. × 32. Courtesy of reference (1).

4

examination of the CSF could lead to the diagnosis of meningeal leukemia, even in the absence of clinical manifestations of CNS disease. Although the proposal was novel then, CSF cytology is now a routine and mandatory procedure in the management of children with acute lymphocytic leukemia.

With increasing leukemic cell invasion the arachnoid becomes packed with cells which extend into the deepest portions as far down as the precapillary arteriole and postcapillary venule levels (Figure 2). These two sites are where the pial-glial membrane fuses with the vasculature to mark the deepest penetration of arachnoid tissue in the parenchyma (Figure 3). Even at this advanced stage of meningeal leukemia, the infiltration of malignant cells remains extraneural, separated from the parenchyma by the pial-glial membrane. It is reasonable to assume that attempts to diffuse lipid insoluble drugs across the BBB and into

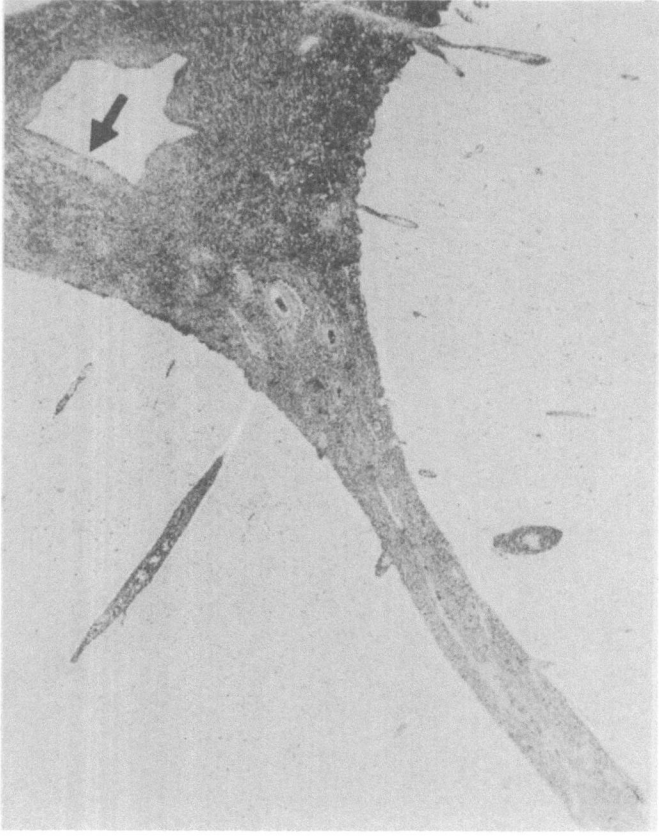

Figure 2. Extensive involvement of entire arachnoid with obliteration of CSF channels and compression of small veins. Large vein (arrow) remains patent, but its wall is infiltrated with leukemic cells. HE. × 33. Courtesy of reference (1).

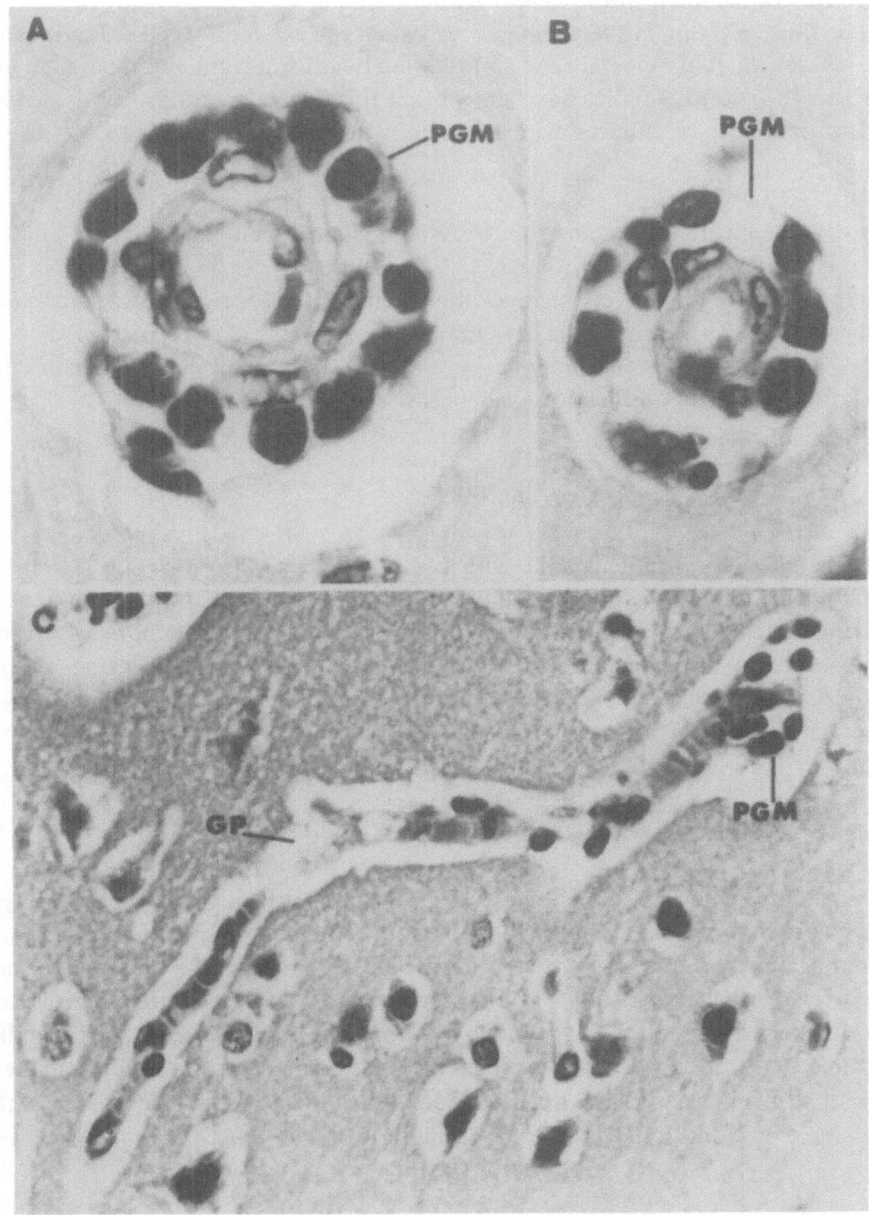

Figure 3. A, B. Leukemic cells in arachnoid at level of precapillary arteriole. The pial-glial membrane (PGM) confines cells to perivascular space formed by the arachnoid. HE. × 1037. C. Capillary in cerebral cortex. A few glial processes (GP) are visible. A precapillary arteriole is surrounded by leukemic cells and the PGM. The surrounding CNS parenchyma is free of leukemia. HE. × 496. Courtesy of reference (1).

the brain would be ineffective, since in most cases leukemic cells are in the meninges rather than in the neural tissue itself (1).

The final step in CNS leukemia occurs when the expanding cell mass destroys the resistant pial-glial membrane and ultimately infiltrates the brain parenchyma (Figure 4). Autopsy studies have shown that this degree of infiltration is present in less than 15% of children with leukemia who died in relapse (1).

Histopathological sequelae, complications and clinical features

There are five phases of meningeal leukemia: 1) destruction of arachnoid trabeculae by infiltrating cells, 2) cranial nerve palsies, 3) obstruction of CSF flow, 4) hypoperfusion encephalopathy, and 5) destruction of pial-glial membrane and direct leukemic infiltration of neural tissue.

Destruction of arachnoid trabeculae

Among children with leukemia with blasts in their CSF on routine lumbar puncture examination, approximately 90% have no symptoms or physical signs of meningeal leukemia (1). This complication of arachnoid leukemia is of critical importance to the clinician since it is only after arachnoid trabeculae are destroyed by leukemic cells that these cells are released into the CSF, permitting a cytological diagnosis of meningeal leukemia (3).

Cranial nerve palsies

All structures entering or leaving the brain must pass through the leptomeninges and can therefore be affected by diseases in the subarachnoid space. Cranial and spinal nerves therefore are particularly susceptible to arachnoid disease and may be affected in at least two ways. First, compression of surrounding vessels and interference with blood flow leading to ischemia within the nerve(s), and secondly, by direct infiltration of the nerve fibers (8–10). Postmortem studies have made it clear that meningeal disease, not leukemic infiltration of brain stem nuclei, is the principal cause of cranial nerve abnormalities (1).

Obstruction to flow of CSF

During the early years of chemotherapy for leukemia, clinical observations revealed that the amount of meningeal leukemia and degree of obliteration of CSF channels were the principal determinants of the hydrocephalus (11). Interference

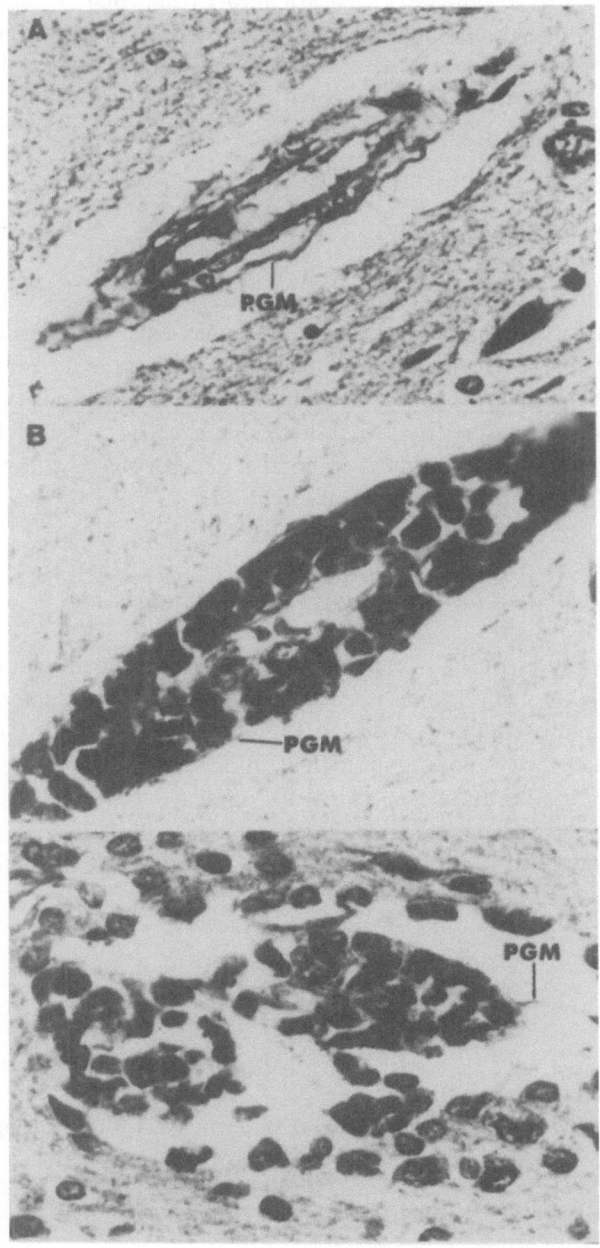

Figure 4. A. Postcapillary venule in cerebral cortex with collapsed (fixation artifact) arachnoid surrounded by pial-glial membrane (PGM). B. Postcapillary venule surrounded by leukemic cells in deep arachnoid limited by PGM. C. Destruction of PGM around postcapillary venule with leukemic invasion of adjacent neural tissue. There is no hemorrhage. Gomori trichrome stain. × 544. Courtesy of reference (1).

with the flow of CSF occurs only after arachnoid trabeculae become swollen with leukemic cells and CSF channels are either compressed or obliterated (Figure 2). Increasing use of intrathecal chemotherapy has been followed by a dramatic decline in the occurrence of hydrocephalus and the concomitant separation of cranial sutures.

Hypoperfusion encephalopathy

Since the arachnoid tissues occupy a finite space, blood vessels within them may be compressed by an expanding mass of leukemic cells. Circulatory impairment due to compressed vessels may follow massive arachnoid leukemia. A number of reports suggest that neurological manifestations can be explained on the basis of a hypoperfusion encephalopathy (10, 12–15). Such neurological deficits, whether temporary or permanent, would depend on such factors as duration and degree of hypoperfusion, and regional collateral circulation.

Destruction of pial-glial membrane and parenchymal invasion

Autopsy studies indicate that leukemic cells directly infiltrate neural tissue only after the pial-glial membrane has been destroyed. This degree of leukemic infiltration probably occurs in less than 15% of all children with this malignancy. Moreover, the severity of arachnoid leukemia seen at the time of autopsy is directly related to the number of previous clinical CNS leukemic relapses (1). Patients with extensive meningeal leukemia have had three to four times as many clinical CNS relapses as patients with no meningeal leukemia detected at autopsy.

References

1. Price RA, Johnson WW: The central nervous system in childhood leukemia. I. The arachnoid. Cancer 31:520–533, 1973.
2. Jaffe RH: Symposium of the recent progress of research in leukemia; pathologic aspects. Arch Pathol 18:763–765, 1934.
3. Schwab RS, Weiss S: The neurologic aspect of leukemia. Am J Med Sci 189:766–778, 1935.
4. Phair JP, Anderson RE, Namiki H: The central nervous system in leukemia. Ann Intern Med 61:863–875, 1964.
5. Fried BM: Leukemia and the central nervous system; with a review of 30 cases from the literature. Arch Pathol Lab Med 2:23–40, 1926.
6. Diamond IB: Leukemic changes in the brain; a report of 14 cases. Arch Neurol Psychiat 32:118–142, 1934.
7. Leidler F, Russel WO: The brain in leukemia; a clinicopathologic study of 20 cases with a review of the literature. Arch Pathol 40:14–33, 1945.

8. Bass MH: Leukemia in children with special reference to lesions in the nervous system. Am J Med Sci 162:647–654, 1921.
9. Hardisty RM, Norman PM: Meningeal leukemia. Arch Dis Child 42:441–447, 1967.
10. Hyman CB, Bogle JM, Brubaker CA, *et al*: Central nervous system involvement by leukemia in children. I. Relationship to systemic leukemia and description of clinical and laboratory manifestations. Blood 25:1–12, 1965.
11. Neis BA, Thomas LB, Freireich EJ: Meningeal leukemia; a follow-up study. Cancer 18:546–553, 1965.
12. Sansone G: Pathomorphosis of acute infantile leukaemia treated with modern therapeutic agents; 'meningoleukemia' and Frolich's obesity. Ann Paediatr 183:3–42, 1954.
13. Joseph MC, Levin SE: Leukaemia and diabetes insipidus; case report with unexpected effect of cortisone. Br Med J 1:1328–1331, 1956.
14. Rosenzweig AI, Kendall JW: Diabetes insipidus as a complication of acute leukemia. Arch Intern Med 117:397–400, 1966.
15. Malter IJ, Gross S, Teree TM: Diabetes insipidus complicating acute lymphocytic leukemia. Am J Dis Child 117:228–230, 1969.

2. Radiation Therapy Methods for Central Nervous System 'Prophylaxis' in the Management of Childhood Leukemias

G.J. D'ANGIO

Introduction

Two principal methods have been employed for irradiating the brain, spinal cord, or both to prevent meningeal leukemia in children. The most common method is external beam irradiation, and the second is the instillation of radiocolloids in the subarachnoid space.

External beam radiation therapy

Irradiation of the central nervous system has been accomplished through a variety of different field arrangements, total doses, and time-dose-fractionation techniques. St. Jude (Children's Research Hospital) in a classic series of studies found 2400 rad to give the best results when doses of 500, 1200, and 2400 rad were tested for this purpose (1). Equally good CNS 'protection' was provided by the administration of 2400 rad to the brain and the spinal cord, or by the use of 2400 rad to the brain supplemented by intrathecal methotrexate. The latter method has become standard therapy in many centers throughout the world. The generally accepted technique is to administer 200 rad on each of twelve successive treatment days using megavoltage units or the equivalent. The portals are arranged in such a way as to include all the meninges (2). This implies the inclusion of the retroorbital space, the paths of the optic nerves, and, for some therapists, widening of the portal at the sacral level to include the lumbar roots.

University of Minnesota investigators used generally similar methods and techniques, and found 1200 rad to be effective in 25 patients given cranio-spinal irradiation. Only one of the 25 developed a CNS relapse (3). This observation, coupled with increasing evidence that 2400 rad, coupled with methotrexate, could produce CNS damage spurred searches for alternate methods of therapy (4). Some investigators, notably those at Memorial Sloan-Kettering Cancer Center eschewed radiation therapy, using intrathecal methotrexate periodically for many months for CNS 'protection' (5).

Children's Cancer Study Group (CCSG) undertook two successive randomized leukemia trials to test various treatment hypotheses (6). The first (CCG-101)

R. Mastrangelo, D.G. Poplack, R. Riccardi (eds), Central Nervous System Leukemia. ISBN 978-94-009-6710-6.
© *1983 Martinus Nijhoff Publishers, Boston.*

examined two radiation therapy modes for CNS 'protection' using 2400 rad; the second (CCG-143) explored whether 1800 rad produced different results. CCG-101 also tested whether 1200 rad given to an extended field that included the gonads, liver, spleen, kidneys and intraabdominal sites affected outcome. Radiation therapy results were compared with those produced when intrathecal metho-trexate (IT MTX) alone was used for CNS 'prophylaxis'. The schemes used in these two studies are summarized in Table 1.

Several different portal arrangements, daily doses, and therapy units were permitted in the protocol specifications. A retrospective review determined whether these non-systematic differences could be correlated with differences in outcome, using relapse in any site, CNS relapse, bone marrow relapse, and survival as end-points.

Extensive multi-variant analyses were undertaken. The analyses included such factors as whether frontal or lateral fields had been used, whether the retro-orbital space had or had not been included in the beam and whether the spinal field had been expanded inferiorly, the daily dose level (which ranged from 120 through 200 rad) and whether kilovoltage or megavoltage units had been used. The same end-points were used in analyzing the patients entered in the second study, where 1800 rad were delivered, and these results were compared to CCG-101 patients irradiated with 2400 rad through comparable fields. The result for low- and high-risk patients, defined as those with initial white blood cell counts below or above $20,000/mm^3$ respectively, are shown in Table 2.

It was found that none of the technical variations, daily dose fractions, or total doses produced statistically significant differences in the CNS or bone marrow relapse rates, or in survival. An exception to the foregoing was the group of children with initial white blood cell counts greater than 20,000 white blood cells per cubic millimeter. Here, bone marrow relapse rates were lowest and survival rates best for those patients given 1800 rad to the brain only plus intrathecal methatrexate. It was concluded that none of the radiation therapy factors analyzed had a major impact on the clinical result (7). This is not to imply that precision radiation therapy and careful dose calculations are not important for the

Table 1

Study No.	Regimen	Code	Description of field and dose
CCG-101	1	2.4 + 1.2 EF	Cranio-spinal – 2400 rad Abdomen and gonad – 1200 rad
	2	2.4/C-S	Cranio-spinal – 2400 rad
	3	2.4/Cr	Cranial – 2400 rad
	4	IT/MTX	No irradiation
CCG-141	5	1.8/C-S	Cranio-spinal – 1800 rad
	6	1.8/Cr	Cranial – 1800 rad

Table 2A. CCG 101/143 Life table estimates (in %) for patients experiencing various end points at 60 months

CNS intensification group	wbc <20,000						
	1 (2.4 + 1.2EF)	2 (2.4/C-s)	3 (2.4/Cr)	4 (IT/MTX)	5 (1.8/C-s)	6 (1.8/Cr)	P-Value*
Number of patients/GP	75	89	109	105	49	46	
Endpoints							
Overall survival	69	80	71	74	78	83	.38
Relapse free survival	65	71	58	51	70	61	.06
Marrow relapse	25	15	31	28	24	23	.25
CNS relapse as first event	8	7	15	33	0	18	<.00

* P values represent overall actuarial comparisons of differences among the regimens by end-point.

Table 2B. CCG 101/143 Life table estimates (in %) for patients experiencing various end points at 60 months

CNS intensification group	wbc >20,000						
	1 (2.4 + 1.2EF)	2 (2.4/C-s)	3 (2.4/Cr)	4 (IT/MTX)	5 (1.8/C-s)	6 (1.8/Cr)	P-Value*
Number of patients/GP	32	37	38	39	14	23	
Endpoints							
Overall survival	47	49	63	44	43	83	.05
Relapse free survival	47	38	55	21	42	65	.03
Marrow relapse	51	53	36	48	59	18	.14
CNS relapse as first event	15	21	14	73	31	20	<.00

* P values represent overall actuarial comparisons of differences among the regimens by end-point.

14

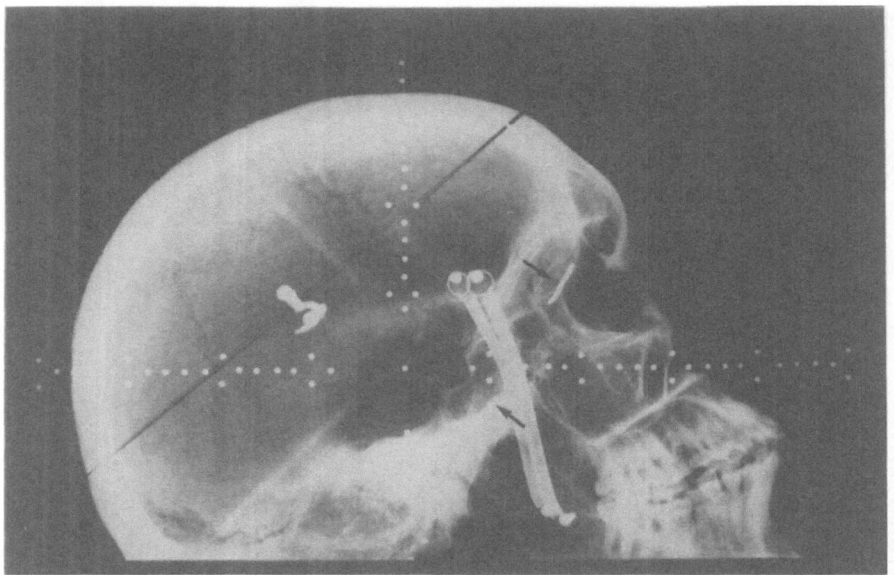

Figure 1. Radiograph of skull (anatomic specimen). The upward pointing arrow indicates a lead marker placed at the inferior recess of the middle fossa. The downward pointing arrow indicates a similar marker placed at the cribriform plate.

individual patient. Every effort should be made to insure accurate beam placement, and coverage of the entire meninges in the portals employed for this purpose. For example, it is important to recall that the cribiform plate lies low in the frontal region, and that the bottom of the middle fossa lies well below the sella turcica (Figure 1).

These results must be interpreted in the light of the regimen 4 patients enrolled in CCG-101. These patients received twice weekly intrathecal methotrexate at a dose of 12 mg per square meter for six doses as their only form of CNS 'prophylaxis'. The meningeal leukemia rate in this sixth group was statistically significantly higher than any of the others; yet, the bone marrow relapse and survival rates have not mirrored this disadvantage over many years of follow-up (7, 8). There is, however, beginning evidence that long-term survival may be worse for the non-irradiated high-risk children (8). This appears to be attributable to repeated bouts of meningeal leukemia, which can be lethal, rather than an increase in the bone marrow relapse rate.

Another system of radiation therapy has been used in Detroit and in Rome (9, 10, 11). Intermittent cranio-spinal irradiation coupled with IT MTX is given to the cranio-spinal axis every ten weeks for three to five years. The methods and the results are reported elsewhere in this volume, but it can be said that this system produces very good CNS 'protection'.

Intrathecal radiocolloids

Radio-active gold (RG) and phosphorous (RP) have been used by different investigators for this purpose. The most experience has been obtained with radio-gold through the work of Metz and Plenert (12–14). They and their coworkers have reported their results in a succession of studies. RG is used in combination with intrathecal methotrexate (IT MTX), the latter being given in doses of 6.25–12 mg/m² for 3 to 15 doses over a period of weeks to 3 years. Doses of RG began with 1 mCi; these investigators are now exploring the use of 4–5 mCi q. 2 wk × 2 for children 2 years of ages or older (15). Metz, *et al* report good results using this method, without any important complications to date. Interpretation of these data is clouded by the fact that IT MTX is also given to all patients. Zanesco and Carli have used radio-phosphorous (RP) for a similar purpose in non-Hodgkins lymphoma patients, but results are too preliminary to be reported (16).

Caution is needed when using intrathecal radioactive colloids, especially if higher doses are contemplated. First, there is the danger of introducing the entire dose in a subdural, extra-arachnoid false space (the 'second sac') that can form after several lumbar punctures (17). Indeed, this caution applies to the repeated administration of any agent given intrathecally. Second, the local dose of irradiation at the puncture site can be quite high and lead to the cauda equina syndrome despite attempts to move the column cephalad, and despite the limited penetration of the rays (18, 19).

Conclusion

Systematic searches for effective, less damaging means of preventing meningeal leukemia are needed. Such searches are encouraged by the good results being reported after different therapies using intrathecal or systemic medications, external beam therapy at various time-dose-fractionation schedules, and their several combinations; and the observation that CNS relapse after inadequate 'prophylaxis' does not inevitably lead to early bone marrow relapse.

References

1. Pinkel D: Five-year follow-up of 'total therapy' of childhood lymphocytic leukemia. JAMA 216:648–652, 1971.
2. Hustu HO, Aur RJA, Verzosa MS, Simone JV, Pinkel D: Prevention of central nervous system leukemia by irradiation. Cancer 32:585–597, 1973.
3. Sharp HL, Nesbit ME, D'Angio GJ, Krivit W: Addition of local radiation after bone marrow remission in acute leukemia in children. Cancer 20:1403–1404, 1967.
4. Duttera MJ, Bleyer WA, Pomeroy TC, Leventhal CM, Leventhal BG: Irradiation, methotrexate toxicity, and the treatment of meningeal leukaemia. Lancet 2:703–707, 1973.

5. Haghbin M, Murphy ML, Tan CC, Clarkson BD, Thaler HT, Passe S, Burchenal J: A long-term clinical follow-up of children with acute lymphoblastic leukemia treated with intensive chemotherapy regimens. Cancer 46:241–252, 1980.
6. Nesbit ME, Robison LL, Littman PS, Sather HN, Ortega J, D'Angio GJ, Hammond GD: Presymptomatic central nervous system therapy in previously untreated childhood acute lymphoblastic leukaemia: Comparison of 1800 rad and 2400 rad. A report for Children's Cancer Study Group. Lancet i:461–466, 1981.
7. D'Angio GJ, Littman P, Nesbit M, Sather H, Hittle R, Ortega J, Donaldson M, Hammong D: Evaluation of radiation therapy factors in prophylactic central nervous system irradiation for childhood leukemia: A report from the Children's Cancer Study Group. Int J Radiation Oncology Biol Phys 7:1031–1038, 1981.
8. Nesbit ME, Sather HN, Ortega J, D'Angio GJ, Robison LL, Donaldson M, Hammond GD: Effect of isolated central nervous system leukaemia on bone marrow remission and survival in childhood acute lymphoblastic leukaemia. A report for Children's Cancer Study Group. Lancet i:1386–1389, 1981.
9. Zuelzer WW, Ravindranath Y, Lusher JM, Sarnaik S, Considine B, Jr: IMFRA (intermittent intrathecal methotrexate and fractional radiation) plus chemotherapy in childhood leukemia. Am J Hemat 1:191–199, 1976.
10. Considine B, Jr, Cook JJ, Zuelzer WW, Ravindranath Y, Lusher JM: Repetitive low-dose radiation therapy for acute stem cell leukemia. Int J Radiation Oncology Biol Phys 2:257–260, 1977.
11. Mastrangelo R, Romanini A, Cellini N, Parenti D, De Renzis C, Riccardi R, Cimatti G, Malandrino R: Intermittent intrathecal methotrexate and fractional radiation (M-IMFRA) plus chemotherapy in childhood leukemia. Tumori 64:607–611, 1978.
12. Metz O, Wieczorek V, Stoll W: Die zerebrale Verträglichkeit der 'Meningosisprophylaxe' mit 198 Au-Goldkolloid an Hand von Liquorbefunden. Kinderärztliche Praxis 12:536–541, 1976.
13. Metz O, Stoll W, Plenert W: Meningosis-'Prophylaxe' mit Radiogold (198-Au) bei der Leukämie im Kindersalter. Dtsch med Wschr 102:43–46, 1977.
14. Metz O, Stoll W: Therapieabschluss bei akuter lymphatischer Leukämie im Kindersalter. Dtsch med Wschr 106:1026–1029, 1981.
15. Metz O: Personal communication.
16. Zanesco L, Carli M: Personal communication.
17. Rogoff EE, Deck MDF, D'Angio GJ: The second sac: a complicating factor in regimens based on intrathecal medications. Am J Roentgenol 120:568–572, 1974.
18. Fuller LG, Rogoff E, Deck M, Galicich J, Ghavimi F, Levitt S, D'Angio GJ: Recent experience with intrathecal radiogold for medulloblastomas and ependymoblastoma: a progress report. Am J Roentgenol 122:75–79, 1974.
19. Sackmann-Muriel F, Schere D, Barengols M, Eppinger-Helft, Braier JL, Pavlovsky S, Macchi GH, Guman L: Remission maintenance therapy for meningeal leukaemia: Intrathecal methotrexate and dexamethasone versus intrathecal craniospinal irradiation with a radiocolloid. Brit J Haematol 33:119–127, 1976.

3. Central Nervous System Prophylaxis for Therapy of Acute Lymphocytic Leukemia

A.M. MAUER, J. OCHS, W.P. BOWMAN, L. CH'IEN,
W. EVANS, R. RAGLAND, R. BERG, L. PARVEY, T. COBURN
and J.V. SIMONE

As an increasing proportion of children treated for acute lymphocytic leukemia are achieving long-term disease-free survival, it has become evident that cure is now a realistic goal of treatment (1). There has been increasing emphasis in recent years, therefore, on the late consequences of the disease and its therapy. These late consequences include possible organ damage, endocrine dysfunction, second malignancies, central nervous system (CNS) dysfunction and psychosocial disorders. This last category may have several factors involved. While the disease produces significant emotional disruption for the patient and the family, there is also evidence that therapy designed to cure the child of leukemia may cause structural alterations of the brain which may, in some children, contribute to the difficulties experienced by the child. In this paper, there will be a historical review of the development of our understanding of this problem. Some data will be presented concerning a retrospective study underway at St. Jude Childrens' Research Hospital to identify the degree and nature of CNS abnormalities found in children who are long-term survivors of the disease and to identify factors which may influence their likelihood. Preliminary information will be presented concerning a prospective study of two forms of CNS prophylaxis with respect to efficacy and late consequences.

Historical perspective

As a greater number of patients experienced longer bone marrow remissions, with improved induction and continuation therapy regimens, proliferation of leukemic blast cells in the central nervous system emerged during the 1960s as a major limiting factor for disease control (2, 3). As control of disease in blood and bone marrow was achieved, more than 50% of the patients were experiencing their first relapse in the CNS (3). Ineffective drug levels were achieved in the cerebrospinal fluid by conventional oral or parenteral administration. The CNS was behaving as a sanctuary site protecting the leukemic blast cells present there until drug resistance occurred. This was followed by a CNS, and subsequently a bone marrow, relapse. A major contribution to the treatment of ALL was the demonstration that the risk of relapse in the CNS could be markedly reduced by treatment with

R. Mastrangelo, D.G. Poplack, R. Riccardi (eds), Central Nervous System Leukemia. ISBN 978-94-009-6710-6.
© *1983 Martinus Nijhoff Publishers, Boston.*

2400 rad irradiation to the craniospinal axis or 2400 rad to the cranium with five doses of methotrexate given intrathecally (4–7). Of even greater importance, was the observation that treatment of this sanctuary area also reduced the frequency of subsequent bone marrow relapse and increased the proportion of patients remaining in continuous complete remission. This CNS phase of the treatment regimen became a standard component of therapy, usually administered immediately following completion of the induction regimen.

In recent years it has become apparent that this form of CNS prophylaxis, while effective, carries some risk of CNS damage. The most important risk has been that associated with irradiation, presumably due to the alterations of vascular permeability to drugs given subsequently. A demyelinating leukoencephalopathy has resulted from the administration of parenteral methotrexate to patients who have had previous cranial irradiation (8, 9). Exact dose relationships are incompletely documented but the risk seems greatest in those patients who have received more than 2,000 rad irradiation followed by methotrexate intravenously in doses greater than 40 mg/m^2/week. Insufficient information is available to determine risks for the development of therapy-related encephalopathy at lesser radiation dose levels. In some circumstances, methotrexate alone appears capable of inducing leukoencephalopathy (10).

Another consequence of cranial irradiation is a mineralizing vasculopathy (11). The likelihood of this irradiation induced change appears to be increased by other risk factors such as the presence of CNS leukemia. The functional consequences associated with this structural change are not known. Additional alterations of the brain have been demonstrated by studies with computerized tomography (12, 13). In addition to mineralization, dilatation of the ventricles and decreased attenuation of white matter have been described. Again, the relationship of these changes to brain function has not been clearly established. In all of these studies, it is impossible to determine the exact risk for the patient receiving cranial irradiation because the studies have been retrospective in nature, relied on autopsy findings or presented small and possibly unrepresentative groups of children treated for ALL. Furthermore, it is hard to determine from these studies what other factors of disease and treatment might contribute to the risk of the irradiation related changes. The need for prospective studies is clearly evident.

Of greatest importance for those treating children with ALL are the functional consequences of these observed changes. A study of neuropsychological functioning of children after CNS prophylaxis with 2400 rad cranial irradiation reported no evident disability. However, the follow-up period was less than two years in the prospective portion of that study (14). An assessment of neurological status and teacher evaluation scores in a group of 22 children, five years after 2400 rad cranial irradiation, also failed to indicate significant functional alteration (15). In other studies of children using psychometric testing given after all therapy for ALL had been stopped, it was found that children who had received CNS prophylactic irradiation under the age of five had reduced IQ scores (16, 17, 18).

Other studies have also indicated the presence of gross neurological abnormalities and apparent learning disabilities in some long-term survivors of ALL who had had 2400 rad cranial irradiation (19, 20, 21).

In light of these observations, attention has turned to alternative methods of CNS prophylaxis that will be as effective as CNS irradiation in the doses mentioned above and yet carry a lesser risk of immediate and late consequences. Intrathecal methotrexate, alone at the time of remission induction, provides ineffective prophylaxis (22), however, when combined with intensive multidrug induction and continuation therapy, it has provided a frequency of first relapse in the CNS equivalent to the standard irradiation regimen (23). Recently, in two studies, the dose of prophylactic CNS irradiation has been reduced to 1800 rad (24, 25). The risk of CNS relapse was equivalent to that when 2400 rad was given for the standard-risk patient but was found to be inadequate for those patients with high-risk features. No studies have been reported as yet to determine the consequences of 1800 rad with respect to CNS alterations. Another proposal of CNS prophylaxis has been the combined use of methotrexate intrathecally and intravenously (26, 27). The methotrexate is given intravenously in large enough doses over a sufficient period of time so that presumably effective drug levels are achieved in the cerebrospinal fluid. Full evaluation of this method must await a longer period of follow-up. It must be emphasized that the efficacy and toxicity of CNS and systemic therapies may be interdependent. For example, the use of intravenous and intrathecal methotrexate (IV, IT MTX), especially in 'standard-risk' patients may allow a somewhat higher incidence of CNS relapse, but this may be offset by superior control of marrow disease (28). To determine effectiveness in disease control as well as the late consequences, it is necessary to observe a group of patients over several years. The final test of any method for CNS prophylaxis must be the likelihood of disease relapse (not only during continuation therapy but also after therapy has been stopped) and the consequences with respect to CNS damage.

Retrospective study of late consequences of CNS prophylaxis

A study was designed to evaluate a relatively homogenous group of long-term survivors of ALL who had received central nervous system prophylaxis which included cranial irradiation with 2400 rad. The objectives of this study were to determine the incidence and type of undesirable long-term therapy-related effects on the CNS, and to see if correlations existed between structural and functional abnormalities and patient characteristics.

Patients to be enrolled on the study were randomly selected at the time of their annual evaluation. A group of 50 patients, which represents almost one-half of the patients eligible, are to be enrolled. Of these, 42 have now completed their evaluation. Patient studies were done without the investigators' knowledge of past clinical course, therapy, or the results of other studies. The evaluation included a complete neurological examination and electroencephalogram, computerized tomographic brain scan, neuropsychological evalution (Wechsler Intelligence Scale (WICS), Wide Range Achievement Test (WRAT) and Selected Reitan Battery), and a review of the chart to determine neonatal course, developmental characteristics, occurrence of CNS infection, seizures, or pneumonia serious enough to require oxygen therapy.

Of the 42 patients, 14 were male and 28 female. Twenty-one patients had received cranial irradiation with intrathecal methotrexate and 21 patients craniospinal irradiation. The median age at diagnosis was four years and eight months and the median time following cessation of therapy was seven years and two months. Twelve patients had had significant clinical episodes including Pneumocystis carinii pneumonia, Cryptococcal meningitis, aseptic meningitis and seizures.

The results of the evaluations to date are as follows: four patients have had disdiadochokinesis on neurological examination; four patients have had abnormal encephalograms with three patients having marked background slowing and one patient having frontal spike waves. On computerized tomographic brain scans, four patients had mineralizing microangiopathy, one mineralizing microangiopathy and leukomalacia, and one leukoencephalopathy.

The neuropsychological evaluation indicated that, taken as a group, the results in these patients were not significantly different from what one would expect in the normative population. The WISC scores showed Full Scale IQ of 100 ± 12.8, Verbal Scale of 98.3 ± 13.6, and Performance Scale of 101.6 ± 14.1. Four patients had Full Scale IQ's in the 70 to 80 range.

The WRAT showed, that as a group, patients did most poorly in arithmetic but overall scores were acceptable in reading and spelling.

Age at diagnosis has been considered to be an important factor for late CNS complications in previous studies. When WISC scores were analyzed for children under and over five years of age at diagnosis, no major differences were detectable between the two groups. When a similar analysis was done for the WRAT, significantly worse performance in arithmetic was found in those patients who were less than five years of age at diagnosis.

When the data from individual children were studied by subscale scores, we found an unusually high incidence of either WISC or WRAT scores below the third percentile. A score below the third percentile indicates almost nonexistent skills in the areas tested and suggests the potential for impairment of academic performance. Seventy-eight percent of these patients were found to have one or more deficient areas and 40 percent had two or more deficient areas. Again, when analyzed by age, younger children fared worse than children older at diagnosis.

One-third of these patients had been referred by various school systems to special remedial classes after cessation of therapy, a factor which does not include private tutors or summer school. Although it is difficult to establish the significance of this finding in a retrospective study, there is the strong suggestion that some of these children may be classified as having learning disabilities.

A review of the variables was made in an effort to identify correlations of such patient characteristics as age and clinical history, abnormal neurological examination, electroencephalogram or computerized tomography scan findings with the neuropsychological evaluation. The majority of patients with abnormal neurological examinations, electroencephalograms, computerized tomographic scans or significant clinical histories were less than five years of age. The majority that did have abnormalities in one of these areas had at least one deficient area on neuropsychological evaluation. An abnormal computerized tomographic scan or clinical history predicted almost one-half of the patients in which two or more deficient areas were found on neuropsychological evaluation. The best single indicator was an abnormal clinical history.

In the conclusions from this study so far, it has been found that about 14 percent of these patients studied retrospectively have had structural brain abnormalities detectable on computerized tomographic scan. In spite of normal Full Scale IQ scores, the majority of these long-term ALL survivors, have had severely deficient areas on WISC or the WRAT. A significant clinical episode, younger age at diagnosis, or an abnormal computerized tomographic scan, characterized those patients more likely to have severely deficient areas in the neuropsychological evaluation.

Prospective study of CNS prophylaxis

One portion of the current St. Jude Children's Research Hospital therapy protocol for standard-risk ALL is the evaluation of two methods of CNS prophylaxis. For the purpose of this study, standard-risk ALL patients are defined as having initial white blood cell counts less than $100,000/mm^3$, no mediastinal mass, no early CNS involvement and lymphoblasts which are E-rosette and surface immunoglobulin negative. All patients have had a standard remission induction regimen including prednisone, vincristine, and L-asparaginase. They have then been randomized to have one of two forms of CNS prophylactic therapy.

One group has received 1800 rad cranial irradiation with intrathecal methotrexate given in a dose of 12 mg/m^2 twice weekly for five doses. The other group was given intravenous methotrexate 200 mg/m^2 as an intravenous push followed by 800 mg/m^2 given over 24 hours. They also received, within one hour of beginning the intravenous medication, intrathecal methotrexate 12 mg/m^2. Blood and spinal fluid levels of methotrexate were monitored for correlation with clinical outcome. Subsequently, the radiation therapy group has been given continuation therapy with sequential changes of drug pairs (6-mercaptopurine and methotrexate, cyclophosphamide and adriamycin, and VM-26 and cytosine arabinoside). This radiation therapy, followed by sequential chemotherapy, has been designated the RTSC group. The patients receiving the IV and IT MTX were given continuation therapy with 6-mercaptopurine and methotrexate with intravenous methotrexate given as above, each six weeks, and intrathecal methotrexate in addition, each 12 weeks. This intravenous and intrathecal group has been designated IV IT.

In addition to a determination of efficacy in prevention of CNS relapse, prospective studies are also being done to evaluate the CNS status. To date, there are 44 evaluable patients in the RTSC group and 47 evaluable in the IV IT group.

With respect to neurological examinations, there have been six patients who developed seizure disorders during maintenance in the RTSC group and two patients who developed seizures in the IV IT group. Sixty percent of the RTSC group had the somnolence syndrome which was delayed in appearance and was clinically milder than has been observed in patients treated with 2400 rad cranial irradiation. On electroencephalographic assessment, 50 percent of the patients were found to have background slowing at diagnosis which resolved within 10 weeks of beginning treatment.

On computerized tomographic scanning, an abnormality suggestive of leukoencephalopathy is defined as a greater than 10 Hounsfield unit difference between the white and grey matter in the frontal horn area. In the RTSC group, three patients had leukoencephalopathy by this definition six weeks after their CNS prophylaxis. One of these has subsequently returned to normal, one continues to have these CT changes over a six month period, and another is too early in the follow-up period. One patient in this group had evidences of mineralizing microangiopathy after one year of therapy. In the IV IT group, seven patients have had this CT finding of leukoencephalopathy six weeks after CNS prophylaxis. It is perhaps notable that despite continuing to receive IV IT MTX infusions, CT scan findings of leukoencephalopathy did not progress and three patients' scores have reverted to normal. An additional four patients developed this change one year after therapy.

Myelin basic protein has been measured in 300 samples by the double antibody radioimmunoassay method. Levels considered increased (greater than one ng/ml) were found in twenty-five patients, only one of whom had the computerized tomographic scan evidence of leukoencephalopathy.

Despite all patients receiving the same dosage of methotrexate, a 3–4 fold range in methotrexate serum concentrations, systemic exposure, and cerebrospinal fluid concentrations has been observed. These interpatient differences are related to the 3–4 fold range in methotrexate systemic (renal and metabolic) clearances measured in these patients. However, there has been no significant correlation between any of these pharmacokinetic variables and the computerized tomographic evidence of leukoencephalopathy observed to date. Longer follow-up will be required to validate these findings and to assess the potential relationship between methotrexate pharmacokinetics and the efficacy of this form of CNS preventive therapy.

Neuropsychological testing has been done with the WISC, WRAT, and selected portions of the Reitan Battery in those children greater than four years of age or upon reaching four years of age. Baseline data alone are available on most patients with only 10 having had follow up examination. It is too early to make any interpretation of these data. The Full Scale IQ in 58 evaluable subjects is 107.

There has been surprisingly little correlation among the various abnormal findings by these techniques, with one exception being abnormal electroencephalograms and the occurrence of seizures.

In general, it is too early to draw conclusions from this prospective study as to which patients will need long-term follow-up for complete evaluation. It does illustrate the importance of prospective studies in evaluating potential risks and identifying factors which may be related to a risk of late consequences of central nervous system prophylaxis and chemotherapy.

Conclusions

As more information has been acquired concerning the late consequences of leukemia and its therapy for central nervous system functioning, it has become evident that much remains to be learned. We have not yet identified all of the factors which, singly or in combination, might influence late central nervous system functioning. We still need more information to determine which, among the various assessment methods, are going to be most sensitive and useful in predicting late functional changes. Of greatest importance is determining which method of CNS prophylaxis is going to provide the greatest efficacy in preventing CNS leukemia and the minimal risk of CNS damage.

Acknowledgement

This work was supported by CNI Grant CA24079, Leukemia Program Project Grant, CA20180, Cancer Center Core Grant, CA21765, Biomedical Research Support Grant, RR05584 and by ALSAC.

References

1. George SL, Aur RJA, Mauer AM, Simone JV: A reappraisal of the results of stopping therapy in childhood leukaemia. N Engl J Med 300:269, 1979.
2. Sullivan MP: Intracranial complications of leukemia in children. Pediatrics 20:757, 1957.
3. Evans AE, Gilbert ES, Sandstra R: The increasing incidence of central nervous system leukemia in children. Cancer 26:404, 1970.
4. Aur RJA, Simone J, Hustu HO, Walters T, Borella L, Pratt C, Pinkel D: Central nervous system therapy and combination chemotherapy of childhood lymphocytic leukemia. Blood 37:272, 1971.

24

5. Aur RJA, Simone JV, Husto HO, Verzosa MS: A comparative study of central nervous system irradiation and intensive chemotherapy early in remission of childhood acute lymphocytic leukemia. Cancer 29:381, 1972.
6. Aur RJA, Hustu HO, Verzosa MS, Wood A, Simone JV: Comparison of two methods of preventing central nervous system leukemia. Blood 42:349, 1973.
7. Report to the Medical Research Council by the Leukaemia Committee and the Working Party on Leukaemia in Childhood: Treatment of acute lymphoblastic leukaemia: Effect of 'prophylactic' therapy against central nervous system leukaemia. Br Med J 351:381, 1973.
8. Price RA, Jamieson PA: The central nervous system in childhood leukemia. II. Subacute leukoencephalopathy. Cancer 35:306, 1975.
9. Rubinstein LJ, Herman MM, Long TF, Wilbur JR: Disseminated necrotizing leukoencephalopathy: A complication of treated central nervous system leukemia and lymphoma. Cancer 35:291, 1975.
10. Meadows AT, Evans AE: Effects of chemotherapy on the central nervous system. A study of parenteral methotrexate in long-term survivors of leukemia and lymphoma in childhood. Cancer 37:1079, 1976.
11. Price RA, Birdwell DA: The central nervous system in childhood leukemia. III. Mineralizing microangiopathy and dystrophic calcification. Cancer 42:717, 1978.
12. Peylan-Ramu N, Poplack DG, Pizzo PA, Adornato BT, DiChiro G: Abnormal CT scans of the brain in asymptomatic children with acute lymphocytic leukemia after propylactic treatment of the central nervous system with radiation and intrathecal chemotherapy. N Engl J Med 298:815, 1978.
13. Enzmann DR, Lane B: Enlargement of subarachnoid spaces and lateral ventricles in pediatric patients undergoing chemotherapy. J Pediatr 92:535, 1978.
14. Soni SS, Marten GW, Pitner SE, Duenas DA, Powazek M: Effects of central-nervous-system irradiation on neuropsychologic functioning of children with acute lymphocytic leukemia. N Engl J Med 293:113, 1975.
15. Verzosa MS, Aur RJA, Simone JV, Hustu HO, Pinkel DP: Five years after central nervous system irradiation of children with leukemia. Int J Radiat Oncol Biol Phys 1:209, 1976.
16. Eiser C, Lansdown R: Retrospective study of intellectual development in children treated for acute lymphoblastic leukaemia. Arch Dis Child 52:525, 1977.
17. Eiser C: Intellectual abilities among survivors of childhood leukaemia as a function of CNS irradiation. Arch Dis Child 53:391, 1978.
18. Goff JR, Anderson HR, Cooper PF: Distractibility and memory deficits in long-term survivors of acute lymphoblastic leukemia. Dev Behav Pediatr 1(4):158, 1980.
19. McIntosh S, Klatskin EH, O'Brien RT, Aspnes GT, Kammerer BL, Snead C, Kalavsky SM, Pearson HA: Chronic neurologic disturbance in childhood leukemia. Cancer 37:853, 1976.
20. Ch'ien LT, Aur RJA, Verzosa JS, Coburn TP, Goff JR, Hustu HO, Price RA, Seifert MJ, Simone JV: Progression of methotrexate-induced leukoencephalopathy in children with leukemia. Med Pediatr Oncol 9:113, 1981.
21. Ch'ien LT, Aur RJA, Stagner S, Cavallo K, Wood A, Goff J, Pitner S, Hustu HO, Seifert MJ, Simone JV: Long-term neurological implications of somnolence syndrome in children with acute lymphocytic leukemia. Ann Neurol 8:273, 1980.
22. Nesbit ME, Sather HN, Ortega J, D'Angio GJ, Robinson LL, Donaldson M, Hammond GD: Effect of isolated central nervous system leukaemia on bone marrow remission and survival in childhood acute lymphoblastic leukaemia. Lancet (June 27):1386, 1981.
23. Hagbin M, Murphy ML, Tan CC, Clarkson BD, Thaler HT, Passe S, Burchenal J: A long-term clinical follow-up of children with acute lymphoblastic leukemia treated with intensive chemotherapy regimens. Cancer 46:241, 1980.
24. Nesbit ME, Robison LL, Littman PS, Sather HN, Ortega J, D'Angio GJ, Hammond GD: Presymptomatic central nervous system therapy in previously untreated childhood acute lympho-

blastic leukaemia: Comparison of 1800 rad and 2400 rad. A report for Children's Cancer Study Group. Lancet (February 28):461, 1981.

25. Henze G, Langermann HJ, Lampert F: Die studie zur behandlung der akuten lymphoblastischen leukaemia 1971–1974 der deutschen arbeitsgemeinschaft fur leukaemie-forschung und behandlung im kindesalter e.V. Analyse der prognosostischen bedeutung von initialbefunde und therapievarianten. Klin Paediatr 191:114, 1979.

26. Moe PJ, Seip M, Finne PH: Intermediate dose methotrexate (IDM) in childhood acute lymphocytic leukemia in Norway. (Preliminary results of a National Treatment Program) Acta Paediatr Scand 70:73, 1981.

27. Freeman AI, Wang JJ, Sinks LF: High-dose methotrexate in acute lymphocytIc leukemia. Cancer Treat Rep 61:727, 1977.

28. Green DM, Freeman AI, Sather HN, Sallan SE, Nesbit ME, Cassady JR, Sinks LF, Hammond D, Frei E: Comparison of three methods of central-nervous-system prophylaxis in childhood acute lymphoblastic leukemiae. Lancet (June 28):1398, 1980.

4. Reduction in Central Nervous System Leukemia with a Pharmacokinetically derived Intrathecal-Methotrexate Dosage Regimen

A Report from the Childrens Cancer Study Group

W.A. BLEYER, C. LEVEL, H.N. SATHER, D.J. NIEBRUGGE,
P.F. COCCIA, S. SIEGEL, P.S. LITTMAN, S.L. LEIKIN,
D.R. MILLER, R.L. CHARD, Jr. and G. DENMAN HAMMOND

Introduction

In 1977, Bleyer and Dedrick proposed a new dosage regimen for intrathecal methotrexate (IT MTX) therapy based on pharmacologic studies which indicated that the primary volume of distribution of IT MTX approximated the extracellular-fluid volume of the central nervous system (CNS) (1). The modified dosage regimen was subsequently confirmed to be less neurotoxic (2), with more consistent cerebrospinal-fluid (CSF) MTX concentrations than dosage based on body surface area (2, 3). Whether or not the altered dose schedule provided enhanced therapeutic benefit remained to be established.

In 1978, the Childrens Cancer Study Group (CCSG) adopted this modified dosage regimen in its CCG-160 series of studies in childhood acute lymphoblastic leukemia (ALL). Since the new therapy was not randomized, a historical evaluation was undertaken to assess its therapeutic effects on prevention of CNS leukemia, continuous complete and hematologic remission durations, and survival. In this report we describe the results of that analysis, which suggest that of all the modifications of preventive CNS therapy applied by the CCSG during the last nine years, the new dosage regimen has been the most effective in preventing CNS leukemia.

Patients and methods

In the period 1976–81, the CCSG enrolled patients on three large randomized trials of therapy for children (defined as < 18 years of age at diagnosis) with ALL. In all, 3241 patients were treated (Table 1). Excluding those patients with CNS leukemia at diagnosis or who failed to achieve marrow remission, 3002 children were treated on one of the three schedules depicted in Figure 2. The systemic treatment programs for these studies have been described in detail elsewhere (4–7).

In studies CCG-141 and CCG-141A, CNS leukemia was defined as symptomatic meningeal leukemia with more than 10 mononuclear cells per microliter in the CSF, or any lymphoblasts provided the CSF cytologic examination was

R. Mastrangelo, D.G. Poplack, R. Riccardi (eds), Central Nervous System Leukemia. ISBN 978-94-009-6710-6.
© *1983 Martinus Nijhoff Publishers, Boston.*

Table 1. CCSG Studies of Childhood Acute Lymphoblastic Leukemia from 1976–1981.

Study	Years patients entered	No. patients entered	Preventive CNS therapies*		
CCG-141	1976–77	877	Cr + IT		
CCG-141A	1977–78	421	Cr + IT		
CCG-161 Low risk	1978–81	405+	IT	Cr mIT	
CCG-162 Ave. risk	1978–81	1123+	Cr + IT		mIT No mIT
CCG-163 High risk	1978–81	415+	Cr + IT + mIT		

* Arrows denote randomizations; Cr - cranial radiation (Cf Fig. 1 for dose), Sp - spinal radiation, EF - extended field radiotherapy, IT - intrathecal MTX, mIT - maintenance IT MTX therapy.

unequivocally positive. In the CCG-160 series of studies, the more sensitive cytocentrifuge technique was applied to the definition: more than 5 white blood cells per microliter in the CSF with cytocentrifuge identification of the presence of leukemic cells.

Statistical analysis of the data from the studies used standard life-table statistics for comparison of remission and survival results (8, 9). Both 'isolated' and isolated plus 'concurrent' CNS relapse rates were analyzed. Isolated CNS relapses were defined as the initial relapse confined to the CNS, and concurrent CNS relapses were those CNS relapses that occurred simultaneously with bone marrow relapse. CNS relapses during a second or subsequent marrow remission were not counted.

In the CCG-160 series of patients, low risk was defined as three to six years of age, inclusive, with an initial white blood cell count below 10,000 per microliter and non-L2 morphology. Average-risk patients were less than three years of age or more than six years old, with a count below 50,000 per microliter; or were three to six years old, with a count between 10,000 and 50,000; or were low-risk patients with L2 FAB morphology. High-risk patients were of any age or FAB morphology with a count above 50,000 per microliter.

Results

The most recent studies, the CCG-160 series, have demonstrated a statistically lower rate of CNS relapse, whether analyzed for isolated occurrences (Figure 2) or isolated plus concurrent relapses (Figure 3). The reduction was statistically significant whether compared with either of the two previous studies or both combined (Figure 4). The comparison with CCG-141A is important because the frequency of IT MTX administration during induction/consolidation was identical in these two studies; only the dose was changed. Overall, the proportion of

CHILDRENS CANCER STUDY GROUP

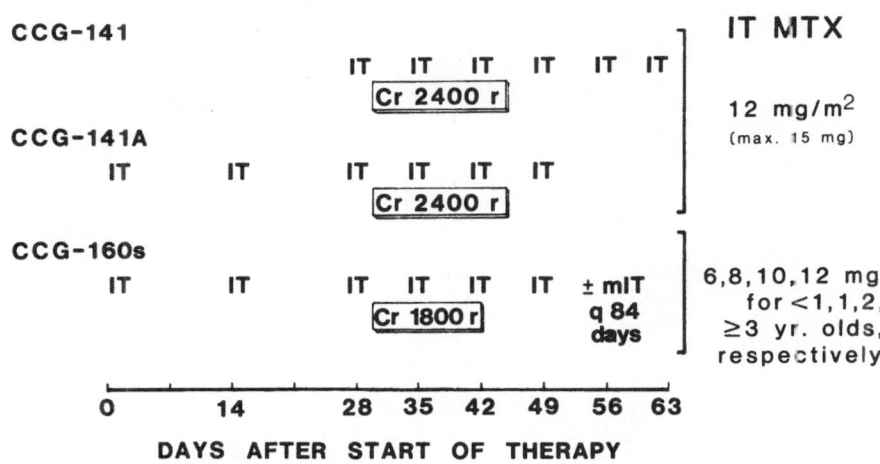

Figure 1. Three strategies of combining CNS radiation and IT MTX to prevent CNS leukemia which were used by the CCSG from 1976–1981 in 3002 patients. In the CCG-141 study, high-risk patients (34% of total number) were randomized to IT MTX on Days 28, 31, 42, 45, 56 and 59 or the schedule shown. In the CCG-160 series, average-risk patients (21% of total) were randomized to maintenance IT MTX (mIT); low-risk patients (58% of total) were randomized to cranial radiation or mIT; high-risk patients (21% of total) were administered mIT (Cf. Table 1).

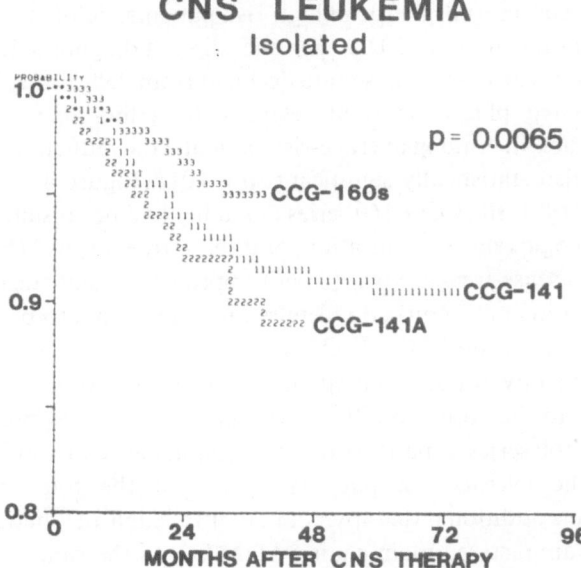

Figure 2. Isolated CNS leukemia on CCG-141, 141A and 160s, as of October 1981.

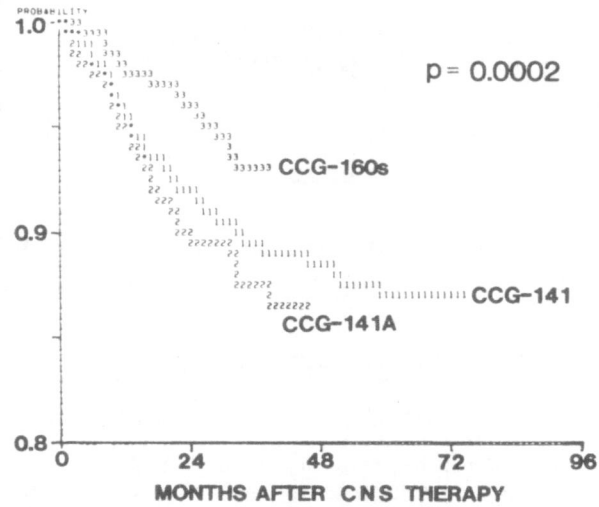

Figure 3. Isolated plus concurrent CNS relapses on CCG-141, 141A and 160s, as of October 1981.

patients experiencing any CNS relapse by three years after completing IT MTX and cranial radiation was reduced from 12.5% on CCG-141A to a life-table estimate of 6.9% on the CCG-160 series (p = 0.0001) (Figure 4).

The reduction was most dramatic in high-risk patients, defined as those with an initial white count greater than 50,000 per microliter at diagnosis. In this group of patients, the three-year CNS relapse rate declined from 23% for isolated relapses, or 27% for isolated plus concurrent relapses, to a life-table estimate of 6% (p < 0.0002) (Figure 4). Among average-risk patients, the reduction was of a lesser magnitude but also statistically significant (p < 0.01) (Figure 4).

As of October 1981, the CCG-160 series of studies had not resulted in improved survival, hematologic remission duration, or disease-free survival (Figs. 5–7), with the p-value for disease-free survival (0.066) approaching statistical significance. The improvement in continuous complete remission appears to be accounted for primarily by the reduction in CNS relapse.

Since the cross-study evaluation used historical controls, other factors that may have contributed to the observed differences were examined. Approximately one-half of the CCG-160 series of patients received maintenance IT MTX, as indicated in Figure 1. The average-risk patients (57.8% of the total number) were randomized to this additional therapy, and all of the high-risk patients (21.4% of the total) were administered maintenance IT MTX. In the randomized phase of this study, there has been no difference to date in the CNS relapse rate (Table 2), either isolated (p = 0.21) or isolated plus concurrent (p > 0.5). IT MTX was given

Table 2. CCG-162: CNS relapse in patients randomized to maintenance IT MTX every 84 days[a]

Time[b] (yr)	No. patients at risk per time interval		Isolated CNS relapse		Any CNS relapse	
Maintenance IT MTX:	M[c]	N[c]	M	N	M	N
1	281	273	1.5%	0.6%	1.7%	0.9%
2	113	113	3.5%	2.1%	3.7%	2.8%
3	5	1	5.0%	2.1%	5.2%	5.2%

[a] Based on life-table estimates
[b] Time from randomization (beginning of maintenance therapy)
[c] Coded regimens - one with and the other without maintenance IT MTX

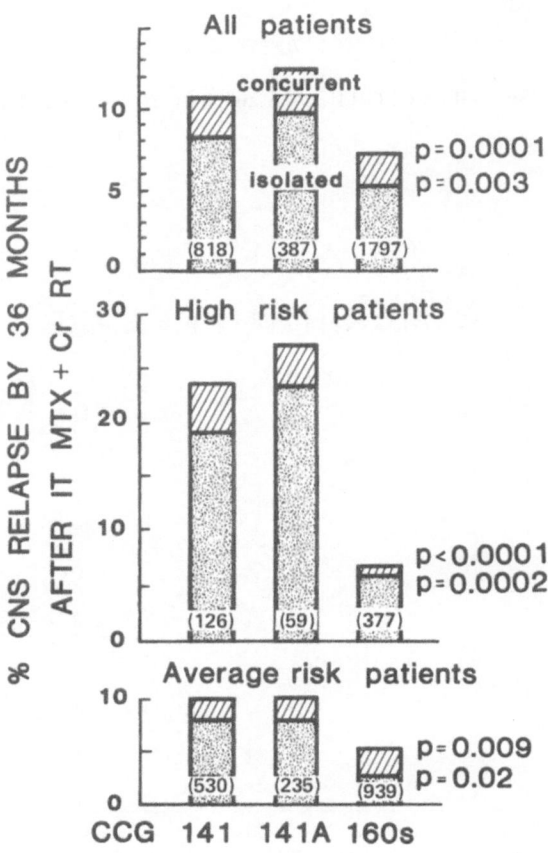

Figure 4. Isolated and concurrent CNS relapse rates by 36 months after IT MTX and cranial radiation (Cr RT). The p-values denote life-table comparisons of CCG-160s versus CCG-141 + 141A.

DISEASE-FREE SURVIVAL

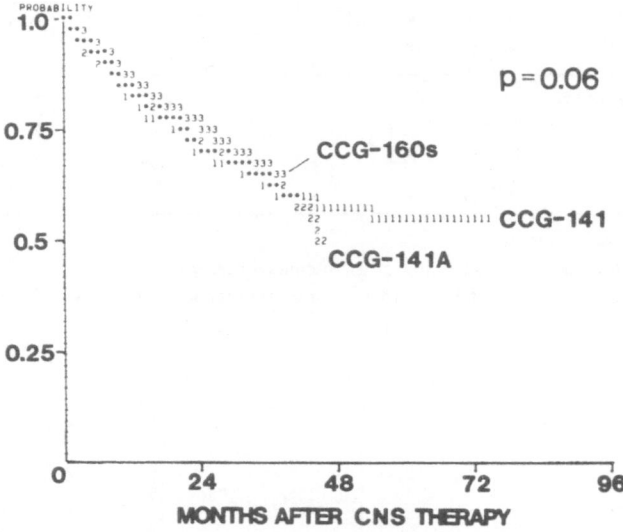

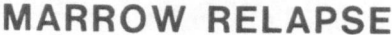

Figure 5. Disease-free survival on CCG-141, 141A and 160s, as of October 1981.

MARROW RELAPSE

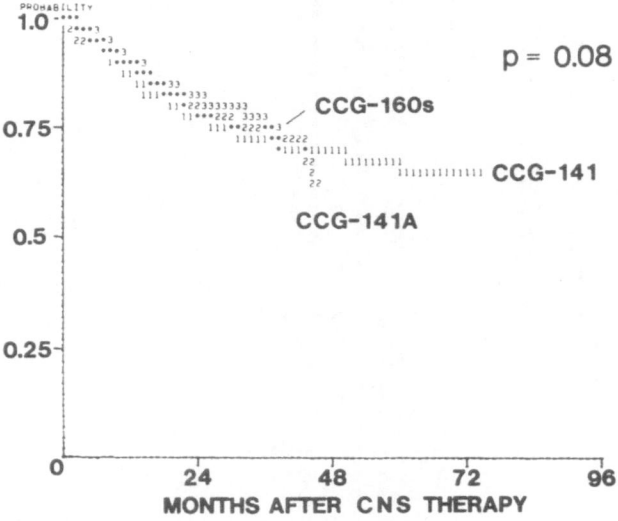

Figure 6. Continuous hematologic remission on CCG-141, 141A and 160s, as of October 1981.

during induction on both the CCG-160 series and the CCG-141A study (Figure 1); CCG-141 withheld IT MTX until consolidation therapy. Induction MTX did not appear to reduce the isolated or overall CNS relapse rate (Figures 2–4). The dose of irradiation was not considered a factor in that this was reduced to 1800 rad for the CCG-160 series, based on the results of CCG-143 (10).

The definition of CNS leukemia was changed somewhat in the CCG-160 studies. The CSF WBC was lowered from 10 to 5 per microliter, and the cytocentrifuge method was routinely applied for CSF cytology evaluation. These changes should have led to an increase in the diagnosis rate of CNS leukemia, not a decrease. Also, lumbar punctures were performed routinely in all patients on the CCG-160 studies, whereas they were performed only when clinically indicated on the prior studies.

Finally, systemic chemotherapy was investigated as a possible contributing factor. Induction therapy was held constant throughout the studies, with vincristine, prednisone and asparaginase given to all patients in each of the studies. Consolidation therapy differed only in the form of CNS treatment. Maintenance therapy on the CCG-160 series depended on the randomization (Table 1). Low-risk patients were randomized to a reduction in therapy with deletion of vincristine/prednisone. Among average-risk patients, one-third received the same therapy as on previous studies, one-third received 'additives'. The latter were pulses of cytosine arabinoside, adriamycin or cyclophosphamide added at monthly intervals to standard maintenance therapy. High-risk patients were

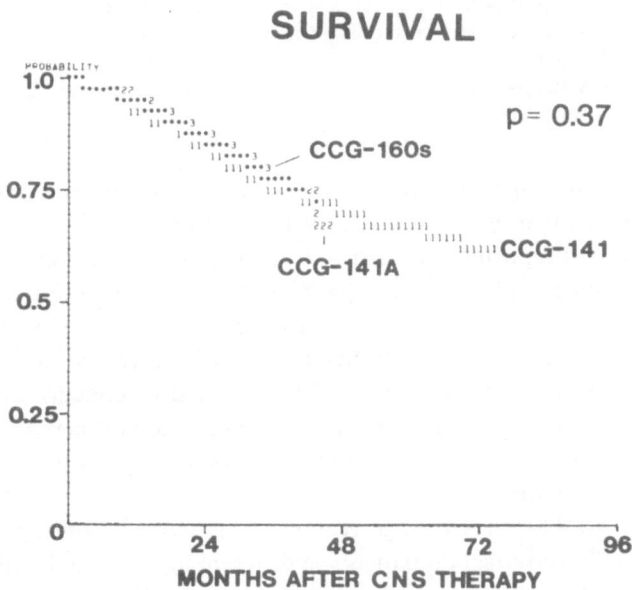

Figure 7. Survival on CCG-141, 141A and 160s, as of October 1981.

34

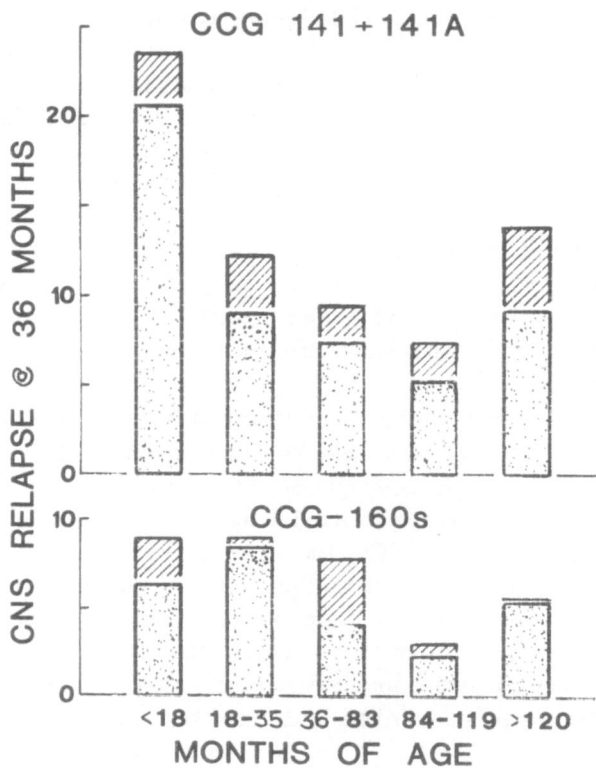

Figure 8. Isolated (stippled bars) and concurrent (hashed bars) CNS leukemia by 36 months after CNS therapy as a function of age at diagnosis. A number of evaluable patients for <18, 18–35, 36–83, 84–119, and >20 months of age were 67, 396, 334, 158 and 250, respectively for the combined CCG-141 and 141A studies, and 90, 364, 750, 218 and 375, respectively for the CCG-160 series.

randomized to the same additives maintenance program or to a cyclical-sequential maintenance regimen in which pulses of POMP (prednisone, vincristine, methotrexate, 6-mercaptopurine), adriamycin and cytosine arabinoside, high-dose cyclophosphamide, and moderate-dose methotrexate were alternated at monthly intervals. As of the time of this report, with a low incidence of CNS leukemia in all regimens, there have been no differences between the various maintenance regimens in the rate of CNS relapse, either isolated or concurrent with marrow relapse. A higher rate of bone marrow relapse has been observed on the cyclical-sequential maintenance treatment for high-risk patients and this regimen has been closed to patient entry.

Since the new IT MTX dosage regimen was derived from age-related pharmacokinetics (3), the effect on patients of different age was analyzed. As observed on previous CCSG studies (11), the incidence of CNS leukemia on CCG-141 and CCG-141A was inversely proportional to age up to 10 years (Figure 8). In the

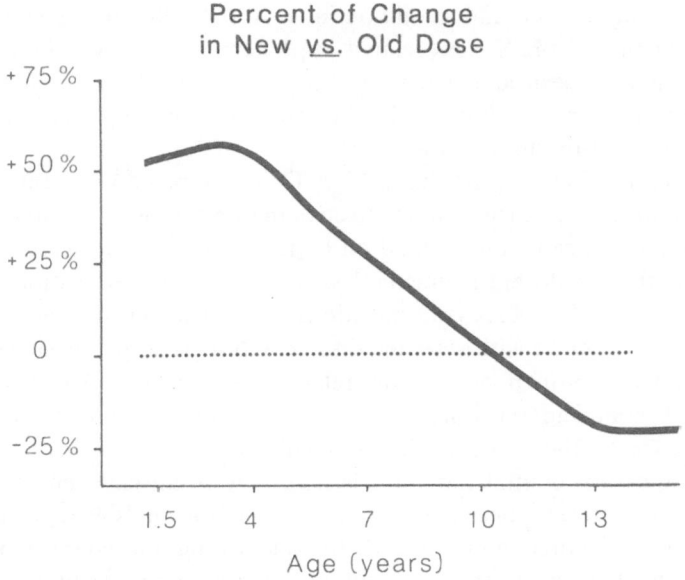

Figure 9. Per cent change in the IT MTX dosage as a function of age with the new dose schedule, used in CCG-160s, compared with the old dose schedule used in CCG-141 and CCG-141A.

CCG-160 series, the reduction in CNS leukemia was most apparent in the youngest patients, with a relatively constant incidence across the age ranges studied (Figure 8). This pattern corresponded to the change in IT MTX dosage, in which the youngest patients received relatively more drug (Figure 9).

Discussion

The Childrens Cancer Study Group (CCSG) incorporated preventive CNS therapy for childhood leukemia in 1972. Since then the CCSG has conducted five large, randomized trials of therapy, only the most recent of which demonstrates a further reduction in the incidence of CNS leukemia. The frequency of routine lumbar punctures and the methods and criteria used to diagnose CNS leukemia were such that if any change in the diagnosis rate were expected on the basis of these factors, the rate should have been increased in the most recent study – not decreased. The data presented here indicates that a revised dosage regimen for IT MTX, based on CNS volume rather than body surface area, was primarily responsible for this improvement. The new dose schedule administers 6, 8, 10 and 12 mg to patients <1, 1–2, 2–3 and ≥3 years of age respectively, regardless of body weight or surface area. Administering IT MTX during induction and/or maintenance therapy did not appear to significantly influence the CNS relapse rate. Reducing the cranial radiation dose from 2400 to 1800 rad has not jeopardized the IT MTX dose-related improvement. The new IT MTX dosage regimen has also been associated with an increase in the projected continuous complete remission rate but not in the estimated three-year continuous-hematologic-remission or survival rates.

These observations suggest that if IT MTX is combined with cranial radiation, the revised dosage regimen is more effective in preventing CNS leukemia than the conventional dosage regimen based on body surface area. Previous studies have shown that the new dosage regimen is less neurotoxic, an observation attributed to more consistent CSF MTX concentrations (1–3). The new dosage schedule does not appear to interact with systemic disease and its therapy, as suggested by the lack of differences in bone marrow relapse and survival. An improvement in continuous complete remission with the new dosage regimen appears to be accounted for by the reduction in CNS leukemia.

Whether or not cranial radiation is necessary in all children with ALL is a separate consideration, one that is not assessed in the analysis reported here. It is under study in the first and last CCSG treatment programs covered in this report: CCG-101 in which one of the four randomized treatments was IT MTX alone and in CCG-161 in which low-risk patients were randomized to cranial irradiation or maintenance IT MTX therapy (Figure 1). The results of the first study, published elsewhere (4), indicate that in general IT MTX alone results in a higher rate of CNS relapse but not in an increased incidence of bone marrow relapse. In that study, patients with isolated CNS relapse after IT MTX alone were apparently more readily salvaged than patients who develop isolated CNS relapse after combined therapy with IT MTX and cranial radiation. In a pilot study for the most recent CCSG therapies, CCG-161P for low-risk patients (age 3–6 years inclusive with initial WBC $< 10,000/\mu l$ and non-L2 FAB morphology), it appears that maintenance IT MTX can be substituted for cranial radiation (12).

In any event, prevention of CNS leukemia is important, particularly in patients administered preventive therapy with combined cranial radiation and intrathecal chemotherapy. The results of the analysis reported here demonstrate that a modification of the IT MTX dosage regimen is associated with a two-fold reduction in overall incidence of CNS leukemia three years after CNS therapy in a three- to five-fold reduction in high-risk patients, whether defined by an initial WBC $> 50,000/\mu l$ or by < 18 months of age at diagnosis.

References

1. Bleyer WA, Dedrick RL: The clinical pharmacology of intrathecal methotrexate. 1. Distribution kinetics in nontoxic patients after lumbar injection. Cancer Treat Rep 61:703-708, 1977.
2. Bleyer WA, Savitch JL, Holcenberg JS: An improved regimen for intrathecal chemotherapy. Clin Pharm Exp Therap 19:103, 1976.

3. Bleyer WA: Clinical pharmacology of intrathecal methotrexate. 2. An improved dosage regimen derived from age-related pharmacokinetics. Cancer Treat Rep 61:1419–1425, 1977.
4. Miller D, Leikin S, Albo V, *et al*: The use of prognostic factors in improving the design and efficiency of clinical trials in childhood leukemia. Cancer Treat Rep 64:381–392, 1980.
5. Miller DR, Leikin S, Albo V, Sather H, Karon M, Hammond D: Intensive therapy and prognostic factors in acute lymphoblastic leukemia of childhood: CCG-141. A report from the Childrens Cancer Study Group. Hemat Blood Transf 26:77–86, 1981.
6. Miller DR: Childhood leukemias. In: Burchenal JH, Oettgen HF (Eds.): Cancer: Achievements, challenges & prospects for the 1980s, Vol. 2, New York: Grune & Stratton, 1981, pp. 319–330.
7. Coccia PF, *et al*: In Press.
8. Mantel M: Evaluation of survival data and two new rank order statistics arising in its consideration. Cancer Chemother Rep 50:163–170, 1966.
9. Peto R, Pike M, Armitage P, *et al*: Design and analysis of randomised clinical trials requiring prolonged observation of each patient: II. Analyses and examples. Br J Cancer 35:1–39, 1977.
10. Nesbit ME, Sather HN, Robison LL, Ortega J, Littman PS, D'Angio GJ, Hammond GD: Presymptomatic central nervous system therapy in previously untreated childhood acute lympho-blastic leukaemia: Comparison of 1800 rad and 2400 rad. A report from the Childrens Cancer Study Group. Lancet 1:461–465, 1981.
11. Bleyer WA: The clinical pharmacology of methotrexate. New applications of an old drug. Cancer 41:36–51, 1978.
12. Coccia PF, Bleyer WA, Siegel SE, Gross S, Sather HN, Hammond GD: Reduced therapy for children with good prognosis acute lymphoblastic leukemia. Blood 56(Supplement 1):000–000, 1981.

5. Central Nervous System Prophylaxis with Intermittent Intrathecal Methotrexate and Fractional Radiation in Childhood Acute Lymphoblastic Leukemia

Y. RAVINDRANATH, K. BHAMBHANI, JOHN K. KELLY,
G. SCHULTZ, I. WARRIER, B. CONSIDINE, J.M. LUSHER
and W.W. ZUELZER

Following the initial studies of the St. Jude group (1), high dose (2400 rad) cranial irradiation plus intrathecal (IT) methotrexate (MTX) or craniospinal irradiation given shortly after remission induction has become the 'standard' form of CNS prophylactic therapy. This form of CNS prophylactic therapy, based on the CNS sanctuary theory, has been widely used and the results obtained with this approach have been discussed by D'Angio (2), Mauer (3), Bleyer (4) and Hardisty (5) elsewhere in this volume.

Conceptual difficulties in accepting sanctuary theory as the sole explanation for the occurrence of CNS leukemia in all cases lead us to develop in 1972 an intermittent form of CNS prophylactic therapy (6). This consisted of periodic administration of IT MTX and fractional low dose (100 r in air) radiation (IMFRA) to the CNS. The results obtained with a chemotherapy regimen which included this form of CNS prophylaxis have been previously shown to be comparable to those obtained with the high dose (2400 rad) initial cranial or craniospinal irradiation (6). Other types of intermittent CNS prophylactic regimens such as periodic administration of IT MTX alone (7) and intermediate dose IV MTX (8, 9) have also been developed. The results obtained with the latter approach are discussed elsewhere in this volume (9).

In any evaluation of the intermittent type of CNS prophylactic therapy, the following questions need to be answered: 1) is the intermittent type of CNS prophylaxis as effective in preventing CNS relapse on therapy as the high dose initial cranial or craniospinal irradiation (with or without IT MTX)?; 2) Is the risk of CNS relapse off therapy higher for patients treated with an intermittent form of CNS prophylaxis?; and, 3) what is the CNS toxicity associated with the intermittent CNS prophylactic therapy?

With these questions in mind we analyzed our experience with the IMFRA regimens. The results of this analysis are discussed below.

Materials and methods

Treatment: The IMFRA regimen evolved from two observations. First, our experience in ALL in the pre-CNS prophylaxis era showed that the first CNS

R. Mastrangelo, D.G. Poplack, R. Riccardi (eds), Central Nervous System Leukemia. ISBN 978-94-009-6710-6.
© *1983 Martinus Nijhoff Publishers, Boston.*

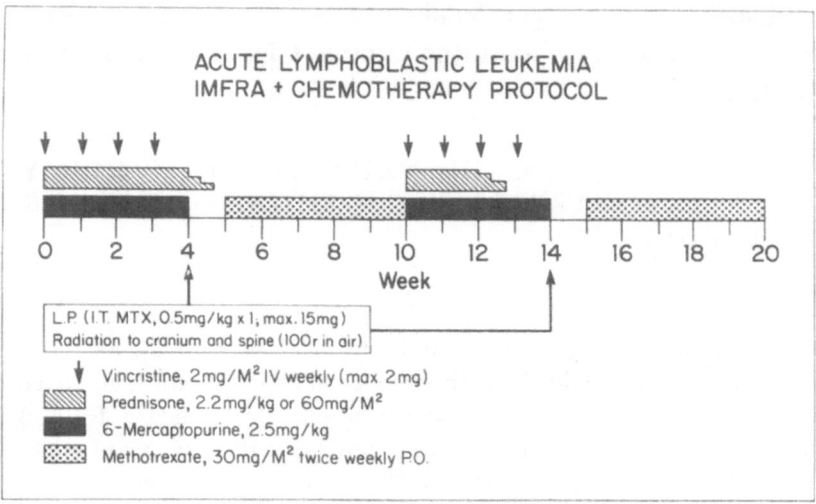

Figure 1. Schema: Radiation is discontinued at 3 years, but IT MTX is continued for the remaining 2 years of systemic chemotherapy.

relapse occurred beyond 12 months of remission in over half the cases, and in some at four or five years of continuous complete remission (CCR), implying a late metastatic spread to the CNS. This suggested that an intermittent form of CNS prophylactic therapy may be more effective. Second, we had previously demonstrated, in established CNS leukemia, that low dose irradiation (100–200 r in air to the CNS) either by itself or following cerebrospinal fluid (CSF) cytoreduction by IT MTX was as effective as higher doses or irradiation (up to 1500 rads) (10, 11).

The IMFRA CNS prophylaxis was incorporated into an effective systemic therapy, as shown in Figure 1. Remission was induced with vincristine (VCR), 6-mercaptopurine (6-MP) and prednisone (Pred) and maintained with alternating cycles of methotrexate 30 mg/M² twice weekly (PO) for six weeks and VCR + 6-MP + Pred for four weeks. IMFRA prophylaxis was started after remission was achieved and was repeated at ten week intervals. Each course of IMFRA consisted of a single IT injection of MTX followed by 100 r in air to each side of the skull (using standard cranial ports) and to the spine. The radiation to the spine was by single port in small children or in two ports for older children. The radiation part of IMFRA was discontinued at three years, but the IT MTX was continued for the remaining two years of systemic therapy. Thus, within the three year period, each child received 15 courses of fractional low dose radiation. The estimated absorbed dose with each course was 160 rads to the skull (80 rads per exposure × 2) and 80 rads to the spine. Therefore, the estimated total radiation dose delivered was 2400 rads to the skull and 1200 rads to the spine.

Patient Material: The study was initiated in February of 1972 and closed for patient entry in February of 1979. Out of 136 newly diagnosed ALL patients entered on the study, 11 died within the first four weeks – most in the early years of the study (Table 1). Remission was attained in 119 of the 125 patients who received a minimum of four weeks of the induction regimen. One hundred thirteen patients were evaluable for analysis of remission duration and survival. The clinical characteristics in these 113 patients are shown in Tables 2 and 3. The sex and racial distributions are as expected. Thirty-nine percent of the patients had a WBC greater than 20,000 at diagnosis, and eight of 113, or 7.0%, had an enlarged thymus at diagnosis.

Table 3 shows the distribution according to the prognostic criteria proposed by the Children's Cancer Study Group (CCSG) with one modification – the patients with a thymic mass are shown as a separate group. The distribution of patients is similar to the data presented by CCSG. Fourteen of the 18 patients in the poor prognostic group, i.e. those with initial WBC greater than $50,000/\mu l$, were males.

Table 1. Total patient material

Total number	136	
Early deaths	11	(8.08%)
	125	
Remission not achieved	6	(4.80%)
Number entering remission	119	(95.2%)
Withdrawn because of CNS relapse prior to initiation of prophylaxis, refusal of CNS irradiation, and poor follow-up in first 6 months	6	
Total evaluable	113	

Table 2. Clinical characteristics

Total number of patients	113
Sex: Male	68
Female	45
Race: Caucasian	97
Black	14
Hispanic	2
WBC at Dx: WBC $<20,000/mm^3$	69
WBC $>20,000/mm^3$	44
Thymic mass	8

Table 3. Distribution of patients according to prognostic groups*

Prognostic groups	Males	Females	Total
Low risk	15	14	29 (25.7%)
(ages 3–7; WBC <10,000/μl)			
Moderate risk	34	24	58 051.3%)
(ages 3–7; WBC 10,000–50,000/μl;			
ages <3, >7; WBC <50,000/μl)			
High risk**	14	4	18 (15.9%)
(all ages; WBC >50,000/μl)			
Thymic mass	5	3	8 (7.1%)
Total	68	45	113

* Prognostic groups are as defined by CCSG (13) with one modification, i.e. the patients with thymic mass at diagnosis are shown as a separate group.
** The differences in the frequency of boys vs. girls falling into this prognostic group were significant by chi-square analysis (P <0.001).

Results

The overall remission and relapse data are shown in Table 4. Forty-six patients relapsed on therapy – 28 in the marrow and 15 in the CNS. One patient had simultaneous marrow and CNS relapse. Extramedullary relapse involving the anterior chamber of the eye was seen in one patient, another developed a chloroma in the orbit. Isolated testicular relapse was not observed. Relapses were more frequent in patients whose initial WBC was greater than 20,000/μl. In all, 58 patients, or 50% of the patients achieving remission, remain alive and in complete remission.

The actuarial survival and remission data obtained by life table analysis is shown in Fig. 2 and Table 5. The complete remission rate for the entire group was 65% at three years and 56% at five years. Both are comparable to most of the published data with a variety of different induction regimens and either an initial single course of CNS prophylaxis therapy or other types of intermittent CNS prophylaxis (1–5, 7–10). The five year remission rate was 80% in the good prognostic group, 69% in the intermediate group, and 24% in the poor prognostic group. For the group of patients with a thymic mass, the five year CR rate was only 12%.

As stated earlier, in 15 of the 113 evaluable patients, or in 13.7% of the patients on study, the CNS was the first relapse site. The actuarial CNS relapse rate is 13% at three years and 19% at five years (Fig. 2 and Table 6). The 13% CNS relapse rate at three years with the IMFRA regimen is not too dissimular from the 13% CNS relapse rate reported by the CCSG with 1800 rad cranial irradiation and IT MTX ×6 (13) and the 10% rate reported by the Cancer and Acute Leukemia Group B (CALGB) using intermediate dose IV MTX and IT MTX ×3 (8).

Further analysis of our data shows that CNS relapse occurred mostly in males (Fig. 3 and Table 7). The male/female difference in the CNS relapse rate (25% versus 8% at five years) was significant with a P value of 0.001. Thirteen of the 15 patients with CNS relapse were males. Of these 13, nine had an initial WBC greater than 20,000/μl, a poor prognostic feature first pointed out by Zuelzer in 1964 (14). The CNS relapse rate for males and females whose initial WBC was less than 20,000/μl was similar. These data identify a special subgroup of ALL patients with a high risk for CNS leukemia, i.e. males with an initial WBC greater than

Table 4. Total case material

Number of evaluable patients	113
Remission deaths	5 (4.4%)
Number at risk	109
Total with relapse	46 (40.7%)
Marrow relapse	28 (25.7%)
CNS relapse	15 (13.7%)
Marrow & CNS relapse	1 (0.8%)
Eye/Orbit relapse	2 (1.8%)
Testes/Other relapse	0
Total relapse with WBC <20,000/μl	23/79 (29%)
WBC >20,000/μl	23/44 (52.3%)
Total number alive in remission	58 (51.3%)

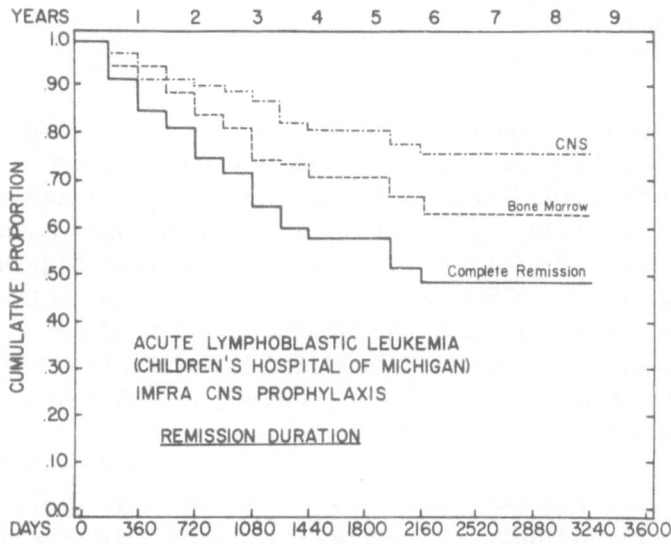

Figure 2. Actuarial remission duration (CNS, bone marrow and complete remission) as calculated by life table analysis.

Table 5. Summary of prognostic factors and remission data

Prognostic groups*	No. of patients	Survival rate**		Remission Rate**	
		3 yrs.	5 yrs.	3 yrs.	5 yrs.
(A) Good risk	29	88%	88%	84%	80%
(B) Intermediate risk	58	84%	66%	72%	69%
(C) Poor risk	18	70%	56%	42%	24%
(D) Thymic mass	8	38%	12%	28%	12%
Total	113	80%	60%	65%	56%

* See table 3 for definition of prognostic groups.
** Survival and remission rates are calculated by life table analysis.

Table 6. Proportion of patients experiencing relapse*

Time (yr.)**	Bone marrow	CNS	Total
1	0.09	0.08	0.16 (113)
2	0.17	0.10	0.25 (85)
3	0.27	0.13	0.35 (79)
4	0.29	0.19	0.40 (65)
5	0.29	0.19	0.44 (50)
6	0.38	0.24	0.51 (39)
7	0.38	0.24	0.51 (28)
8	0.38	0.24	0.51 (24)
9	0.38	0.24	0.51 (19)

* Based on life table analysis.
** Time from diagnosis.
Numbers in parenthesis are patients at risk.

$20,000/\mu l$. In this subgroup of patients, IMFRA CNS prophylaxis was inadequate, and this apparently is the explanation for the somewhat high rate of CNS relapse seen with IMFRA CNS prophylaxis compared to other studies. The influence of initial white count on the incidence of CNS relapse is illustrated even more dramatically in Table 8. As shown here, patients in the poor prognostic group as defined by CCSG, i.e. those with initial WBC greater than $50,000/\mu l$, experienced an extraordinarily high incidence of CNS relapse, a fact recently pointed out by Nesbit *et al* (13). It is interesting to note that 14 of the 18 patients in this group were males and seven had CNS relapse as the first event including the one with simultaneous BM and CNS relapse.

The course after cessation of therapy at five years in the IMFRA group is shown in Table 9. So far, treatment has been stopped in 40 IMFRA treated patients. In five, treatment was stopped at three years. Three patients refused all or part of the treatment at three years; two additional patients moved to other areas, and in them treatment was stopped at three years of CCR by their present

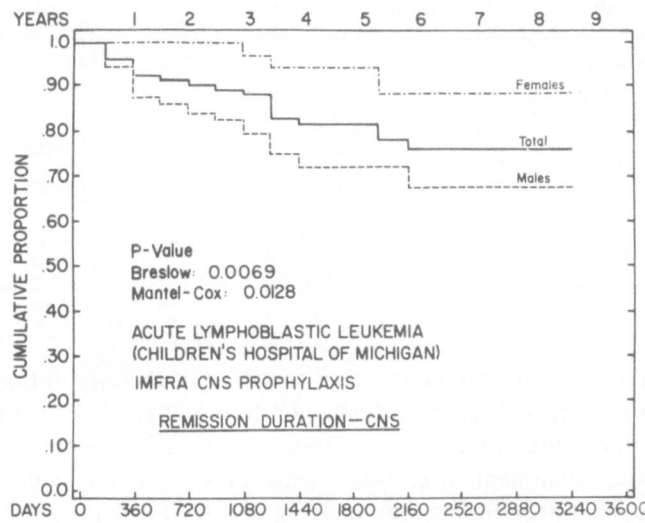

Figure 3. Actuarial curves of CNS remission duration.

Table 7. Incidence of CNS relapse

	Males	Females	P value	Total
Total	68	45		113
Number with relapse	13	2	0.006	15 (13.3%)
WBC <20,000/μl	43	36		79
Number with relapse	4 (9.3%)	2 (5.6%)	0.23	6 (7.6%)
WBC >20,000/μl	25	9		34
Number with with relapse	9 (36%)	0	<0.001	9 (26.5%)

Table 8. Proportion of patients experiencing CNS relapse*

Prognostic group	Time (in months) from diagnosis					
	12	24	36	48	60	72
Good (N = 29)	0.03	0.07	0.11	0.11	0.17	0.17
Intermediate (N = 58)	0.0	0.02	0.04	0.09	0.09	0.15
Poor (N = 18)	0.26	0.26	0.44	0.61	0.61	0.61
Thymic mass (N = 8)	0.12	0.12	0.12	0.12	0.12	0.12

* By life table analysis

Table 9. Course after cessation of therapy

Number off-therapy	40
Follow-up off-therapy	
Median	2 years
Range	1 mo.–4 yrs.
Number with relapse	5 (12.5%)
Marrow	3
CNS	1
Marrow & CNS	1

physician. The median observation post cessation of therapy in this group of 40 patients is two years with a range of one month to four years. Five, or 12.5%, have relapsed so far. Three of the five relapses occurred in the three patients who refused further treatment after three years of CR. Three patients had bone marrow relapse, one simultaneous marrow and CNS relapse, and one isolated CNS relapse. No relapses have occurred after six years of complete remission. Thus, the post therapy course in these patients appears to be similar to that for patients who received high dose CNS irradiation early in remission for CNS prophylaxis. Life table analysis indicates that 48% of the patients entered may be expected to be in CR six years from diagnosis (Figure 2).

The CNS toxicity observed with IMFRA CNS prophylaxis was minimal (Table 10). Arachnoiditis related to IT MTX was seen in nearly 50% of the patients, requiring dosage adjustment. Long-term CNS toxicity was noted in only two patients; both developed seizure disorders within the first year of systemic therapy. In one, seizures started after the first course of IMFRA and in the other at ten months of CCR. CT scans of the brain were normal in these two patients. CAT scans of the brain were also performed in 27 of the 40 patients off therapy and these were normal. No cases of mineralizing angiopathy or brain atrophy were seen. We have not performed any systematic psychometric testing and thus cannot comment on subtle learning disabilities in our patients.

A comment is now in order regarding the three cases in whom we reported on the development of morphologically different leukemia at the time of relapse – one case of JCML and two cases of AML (15). No other examples of morphologic shift were seen. It is possible that these are therapy related and the low dose radiation was contributory. However, such cases have been described with other forms of CNS prophylactic therapy (16) and could as well be from chance occurrence.

Discussion

The data presented above show that the IMFRA therapy is an effective form of

CNS prophylactic therapy. The overall results are comparable to the published results obtained with regimens utilizing high dose initial cranial or craniospinal irradiation. A somewhat higher actuarial rate of CNS relapse was noted in this study. CNS relapse was more frequent in boys than in girls. However, this increased risk of CNS relapse in boys was restricted to those with a high initial WBC (greater than 20,000/μl). The marrow and CNS relapse rates for males and females with an initial WBC less than 20,000/μl were similar.

Analysis of our data utilizing the prognostic groups as defined by the CCSG shows results comparable to that recently reported by CCSG, viz. patients in the poor prognostic group (those with initial WBC greater than 50,000/μl) experience a high rate of CNS relapse. Interestingly, 14 of 18 patients in this group were boys, and 7 of 14 had CNS relapse as first event. This difference in the CNS relapse rate seems to account for the male/female difference in the complete remission rates on therapy in our study (data not shown). No significant differences in either CNS, marrow or complete remission rates were noted between boys and girls in the good or intermediate prognostic groups using CCSG criteria.

The course after cessation of therapy in the IMFRA treated group compares favorably with the results recently reported by the St. Jude group (17, 18). Five of 40 patients (12%) who had therapy discontinued relapsed. One patient had isolated CNS relapse, one patient had simultaneous CNS and marrow relapse and the remaining three had marrow relapse.

These data show that IMFRA CNS prophylaxis is effective in preventing CNS relapse both on and off therapy. Patients receiving this type of intermittent CNS prophylaxis are at no higher risk of relapse after cessation of therapy. CT scan evaluation of patients in whom therapy was discontinued did not show any significant abnormalities, suggesting that this form of CNS prophylactic therapy may be less toxic to the CNS. However, detailed psychometric studies are necessary to confirm this.

Acknowledgments

The authors gratefully acknowledge the help of Patricia Karwoski and Cynthia Tanner in the preparation and typing of this manuscript.

References

1. Aur RJA, Simme J, Husto HO, Walter T, Borella L, Pratt C, Pinkel D: Central Nervous System therapy and continuation chemotherapy of childhood acute lymphoblastic leukemia. Blood 37:272–281, 1971.
2. D'Angio GJ: Central Nervous System prophylaxis for acute lymphoblastic leukemia of childhood: radiation therapy factors. This issue.
3. Mauer AM: Central nervous system prophylaxis: the St. Jude experience. This issue.

48

4. Bleyer WA: Central Nervous System prophylaxis: Children's Cancer Study Group results. This issue.
5. Hardisty RM: Prophylaxis of central nervous system leukemia: recent British experience. This issue.
6. Zuelzer WW, Ravindranath Y, Lusher JM, Sarnaik S, Considine B: IMFRA (Intermittent Intrathecal Methotrexate and Fractional Irradiation) plus chemotherapy in childhood acute leukemia. Am J Hematology 1:191–199, 1976.
7. Haghbin M, Murphy ML, Tan CC, Clarkson BD, Thaler HT, Passe S, Burchenal J: A long term clinical follow-up with acute lymphoblastic leukemia treated with intensive chemotherapy regimes. Cancer 46:241–282, 1980.
8. Sinks L, Wang JJ, Freeman AI: The treatment of primary childhood acute lymphocytic leukemia with intermediate dose Methotrexate. Modern trends in human leukemia IV. (Latest results in clinical biological research including pediatrics-oncology). Neth R, Gallo RC, Graf T, Mannweiler K, Winkler K (eds), Springer Verlag, 1981, p 107.
9. Moe P: Central nervous system prophylaxis with intermediate dose methotrexate. This issue.
10. Haghbin M, Zuelzer WW: A long term study of cerebrospinal leukemia. J Pediat 67:23–28, 1965.
11. Cook J, Considine B: Low dose radiation therapy for leukemic involvement of the central nervous system. Radiology 104:649–652, 1972.
12. Coccia P, Sather H, Nesbit M, Weiner J, Donaldson M, Hittle R, Ortega J, Hammond D: Interrelationship of initial WBC, age and sex in predicting prognosis in childhood acute lymphoblastic leukemia (Abstr. #214). Proc Am Hematol, 1976, p 125.
13. Nesbit ME, Sather HN, Robison LL, Ortega J, Littman PS, D'Angio GJ, Hammond GD: Presymptomatic central nervous system therapy in previously untreated childhood acute lymphoblastic leukemia: comparison of 1800 rad and 2400 rad. A report for Children's Cancer Study Group. Lancet 1:461–466, 1981.
14. Zuelzer WW: Implications of long term survival in acute stem cell leukemia of childhood treated with comparable cyclic therapy. Blood 26:477–494, 1964.
15. Ravindranath Y, Inoue S, Considine B, Lusher JM, Zuelzer WW: New leukemia in the course of therapy of acute lymphoblastic leukemia. Am J Hematol 5:211–223, 1978.
16. Mosijczuk AD, Ruymann FR: Second malignancy in acute lymphocytic leukemia. Review of 33 cases. Am J Dis Child 135:313–316, 1981.
17. George SL, Aur RJA, Mauer AM, Simme JV: A reappraisal of the results of stopping therapy in childhood leukemia. New Eng J Med 300:269–273, 1979.
18. Ravindranath Y, Soorya DJ, Schultz GE, Lusher JM: Long term survivors of acute lymphoblastic leukemia – risk of relapse after cessation of therapy. Med Ped Oncol 9:209–218, 1981.

6. Intermittent Intrathecal Methotrexate and Fractional Radiation plus Chemotherapy in Childhood Lymphoblastic Leukemia

R. MASTRANGELO, R. RICCARDI, R. MALANDRINO
and A. ROMANINI

Early prophylactic irradiation of the Central Nervous System (CNS) has greatly improved the prognosis in children with Acute Lymphoblastic Leukemia (ALL) (1).

Cranial irradiation with 2400 rad or, more recently, 1800 rad in conjunction with Intrathecal Methotrexate (IT MTX) is currently the most widely used preventive therapy for CNS leukemia (2–3). The rationale for this approach is based on the assumption that leukemic cells are present in the CNS at the time of diagnosis and that radiotherapy can eliminate the lymphoblasts protected from therapeutic agents from the blood-brain barrier. However, meningeal leukemia may not be only present at diagnosis but theoretically can arise from subsequent spread from the bone marrow at later stages of the disease.

Based on this possibility, a protocol was devised by Zuelzer (4) some years ago which included intermittent low dose radiation both to the cranial vault and to the spine as a method of preventing meningeal leukemia. The present report discusses the results of a clinical study performed using a similar treatment approach.

Materials and methods

Figure 1 shows the ALL protocol utilized in this study. Following remission and at each cycle of reinduction, CNS prophylaxis was performed administering 100 rad from a ^{60}Co unit to each side of the skull and to the spine. Lumbar punctures were performed prior to each dose of radiation. CSF samples were examined for cell count and morphology by cytocentrifuge analysis. The diagnosis of meningeal leukemia was based on the presence, on a cytocentrifuge preparation, of leukemic cells in the CSF. At the time of spinal tap, a single administration of MTX (0.4 mg/kg, maximum dose 12 mg) was given. Systemic induction chemotherapy consisted of Vincristine, Prednisone and 6-MP and was followed by daily 6-MP and biweekly oral MTX as maintenance. This induction-maintenance cycle was repeated every ten weeks for a total of 36 months.

Sixty-one consecutive patients were treated between March '74 and May '81 at the Clinica Pediatrica of the Catholic University of Rome. Of these, 35 were high risk patients, as judged by WBC above 20,000/mm^3 (n = 28), mediastinal mass

R. Mastrangelo, D.G. Poplack, R. Riccardi (eds), Central Nervous System Leukemia. ISBN 978-94-009-6710-6.
© *1983 Martinus Nijhoff Publishers, Boston.*

50

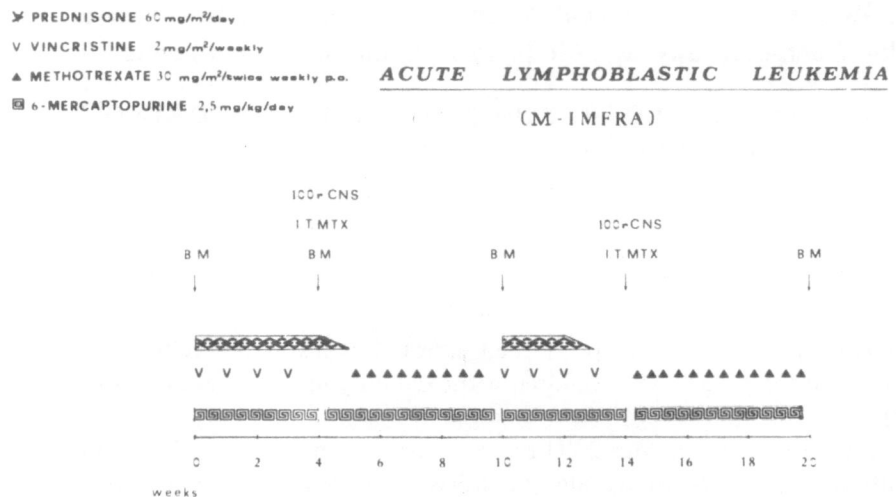

Figure 1. M-IMFRA protocol-treatment schema.

(n = 10) and age under 18 months (n = 4) or over 12 years (n = 8).

Fourteen of the 61 patients were studied with axial computerized tomography (CT) after completion of the entire three years of this modified IMFRA protocol. At the time of CT their age ranged from 11 months to 14 years at diagnosis and the interval between diagnosis and CT ranged from 36 to 49 months. CT was performed utilizing a Siemens Head Scanner model Sireton 2000. Evaluation of the CT findings was carried out by a neuroradiologist who had no prior clinical information about the patients. Ventricular size was quantitatively assessed by linear measurement technique (5). Quantitative evaluation of white-matter density (attenuation coefficient) was also performed. Complete neurologic evaluation of ALL patients was done by a neurologist who also had no prior knowledge of the patients.

Results

Of the initial 61 patients, 2 did not achieve complete remission and 4 died in complete remission: three from viral pneumonia and one from viral hepatitis. Two had CNS leukemia at diagnosis, one patient developed toxic hepatitis which prevented additional methotrexate treatment and one patient was lost to follow-up. The evaluation of remission duration was based on the remaining 51 patients with a period of observation up to 86 months. Of the 51 patients, 14 have relapsed, 10 in the bone marrow (6 low risk and 4 high risk) and 4 in the CNS (4 high risk patients).

Figure 2 shows the actuarial curve with 63% of the patients surviving free of

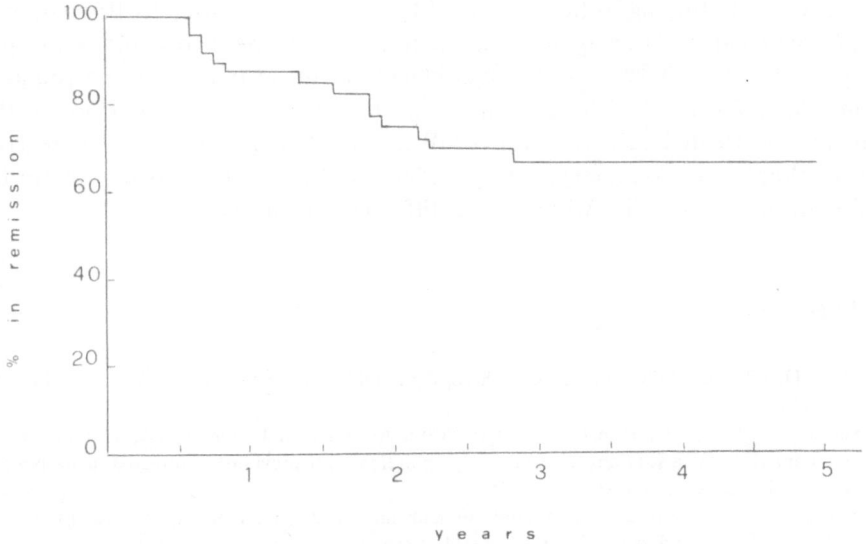

Figure 2. Duration of complete remission of children with ALL treated according to M-IMFRA protocol.

disease at 5 years with a median of 39 months. CNS relapse occurred in 8% of the patients.

Of the 14 patients initially evaluated by CT scans, two developed CNS leukemia shortly after the CT scan was done and could not be evaluated. Of the remaining 12 patients, five showed one or two abnormal CT scan findings. Two patients showed ventricular dilatation and three both ventricular dilatation and subarachnoid space dilatation.

Discussion

Our results compare favorably with those achieved when initial CNS irradiation with 2400 rad or 1800 rad is used in conjunction with IT MTX. The incidence of CNS relapse as well as the remission duration are similar to those reported by other institutions where the 'standard' CNS prophylaxis is adopted (2–3). At the same time the M-IMFRA protocol appears to be simple, with limited traumatic and toxic side effects.

One of the aims of the protocol was to minimize the treatment sequelae related to meningeal leukemia prophylaxis. We found CT abnormalities in about 40% of our asymptomatic patients after cessation of the treatment. Ventricular dilatation and subarachnoid space dilatation were the only CT abnormalities noted. Intracerebral calcifications and decreased attenuation coefficient, findings described in other reports, were not observed in our patients (6).

Our CT scan findings differ considerably from those reported by Ravindranath *et al.* (see Chapter 5) using a similar treatment protocol. Those authors studied 27 patients with CT scans following virtually identical treatment and found no abnormal CT findings. The only difference between that study and ours is that patients we treated received oral 6-MP as maintenance therapy and received orthovoltage rather than megavoltage radiation. Whether the explanation for this CT scan discrepancy lies within these differences is unclear.

References

1. Pinkel D: Five year follow up of 'total therapy' of childhood lymphocytic leukemia. JAMA 216: 648, 1971.
2. Nesbit ME, Sather H, Robison LL, Donaldson M, Littman P, Ortega JA, Hammond GD: Sanctuary therapy: a randomized trial of 724 children with previously untreated acute lymphoblastic leukemia. Cancer Res 42:674, 1982.
3. Mauer AM: Therapy of acute lymphoblastic leukemia in childhood. Blood 56:1–10, 1980.
4. Zuelzer WW, Ravindranath Y, Lusher JM, Sarnaik S, Considine B: IMFRA (intermittent intrathecal methotrexate and fractional radiation) plus chemotherapy in childhood leukemia. Am J Hemat 1:191, 1976.
5. Enzmann DR, Lane B: Cranial computed tomography findings in anorexia nervosa. J Comput Assist Tomography 1:410, 1977.
6. Peylan-Ramu N, Poplack DG, Pizzo PA, Adornato BT, DiChiro G: Abnormal CT scans of the brain in asymptomatic children with acute lymphocytic leukemia after prophylactic treatment of the central nervous system with radiation and intrathecal chemotherapy. N Engl J Med 298: 815, 1978.

7. Prophylaxis of Central Nervous System Leukaemia: British Experience, 1970–80

R.M. HARDISTY

In the first of the series of therapeutic trials in acute lymphoblastic leukaemia of childhood (UKALL I) conducted for the Medical Research Council in the United Kingdom, one of the variables was 'prophylactic' treatment against central nervous system (CNS) leukaemia. In view of the overwhelming evidence for the efficacy of such treatment (1, 2), all patients entered to subsequent trials have received some form of CNS prophylaxis. This report compares the results to date of the various prophylactic regimes used in UKALL trials I–V, to which patients were entered between 1970 and 1979.

Patients and methods

The dates of entry to the various trials and the CNS irradiation dosages are shown in Table 1. Details of the radiotherapy and chemotherapy schedules have been previously published (2–5), except for UKALL IV; this was confined to patients with initial leucocyte counts over $20 \times 10^9/l$, who were randomized to induction with COAP or with vincristine and prednisolone, and then to intermittent or continuous maintenance regimes. UKALL V was designed for patients with leucocyte counts not exceeding $20 \times 10^9/l$ at diagnosis. Chemotherapy was stopped, in patients in complete remission, after either six or twelve 12-week maintenance cycles in UKALL I, and after eight or twelve cycles in subsequent trials.

Patients in UKALL I who received CNS irradiation also had eleven doses of intrathecal methotrexate (10 mg/m^2) between weeks 17 and 55; all other patients on CNS prophylaxis (except those in UKALL II who received 2400 rads to the spinal cord, but no intrathecal methotrexate) had 5 weekly doses of intrathecal methotrexate over a period embracing the radiotherapy. In UKALL V, most patients were non-randomly allocated to one of three cranial radiation schedules: 2400 rad in 15 fractions, 2400 rad in 12 fractions, or 2100 rad in 7 fractions. Details of fractionation were not standardized in the remaining patients in this and other trials, but the total dose was usually given in $2\frac{1}{2}$–$5\frac{1}{2}$ weeks. Supervoltage apparatus was used in the great majority of cases, and cranial irradiation was given by opposing lateral fields designed to include the posterior orbit.

R. Mastrangelo, D.G. Poplack, R. Riccardi (eds), Central Nervous System Leukemia. ISBN 978-94-009-6710-6.
© *1983 Martinus Nijhoff Publishers, Boston.*

The present analyses are confined to patients aged less than 14 years at diagnosis of leukaemia, who were in complete remission at week 12 (i.e. after the end of prophylactic radiotherapy). Follow-up data on all trials to December 31st 1980 have been analyzed by life-table methods as described by Peto *et al* (6).

Results

Early CNS leukaemia. Of the 134 patients not in complete remission at week 12 (Table 1), 14 had already developed CNS leukaemia, either at the time of initial diagnosis or during the induction phase. This represents an overall incidence of 0.3% (3/1060) for patients with presenting leucocyte counts of $20 \times 10^9/l$ and below, and 3.0% (11/369) for those with higher counts. Of these 14 patients, 7 survived less than 12 months, 4 between one and two years, and only 3 more than two years.

CNS relapse. All forms of CNS prophylaxis significantly reduced the CNS relapse rate (Figures 1 and 2), low-dose spinal irradiation and intrathecal methotrexate appearing marginally better, and high-dose spinal irradiation slightly less effective, than cranial irradiation with intrathecal methotrexate alone. These trends were apparent for both high- and low-count patients, but achieved statistical significance only for the latter group (Table 2). In UKALL I, no significant difference has yet emerged between the three fractionation schedules for cranial irradiation, though the CNS relapse rate appears to be somewhat lower in the group receiving the largest number of fractions than in the remainder (Figure 3).

Bone-marrow relapse. For the purposes of the present analysis, the duration of

Table 1. UKALL I–V: Case material NR, patients not in complete remission at 12 weeks and excluded from the present analyses.

UKALL	Entry	Radiotherapy (rads)				NR (%)
		NIL	CR 2400 only	Cr 2400 Sp 1000	Cr 2400 Sp 2400	
I	1970–71	81	—	72	—	23 (13)
II	1972–73	—	72	108	74	24 (8)
III	1973–75	—	291	—	—	24 (8)
IV (>20K)	1975–77	—	163	—	—	36 (18)
V (≤20K)	1976–79	—	494*	—	—	27 (5)
Total		81	1020	180	74	134 (9)

* Including 121 receiving Cr 2100.

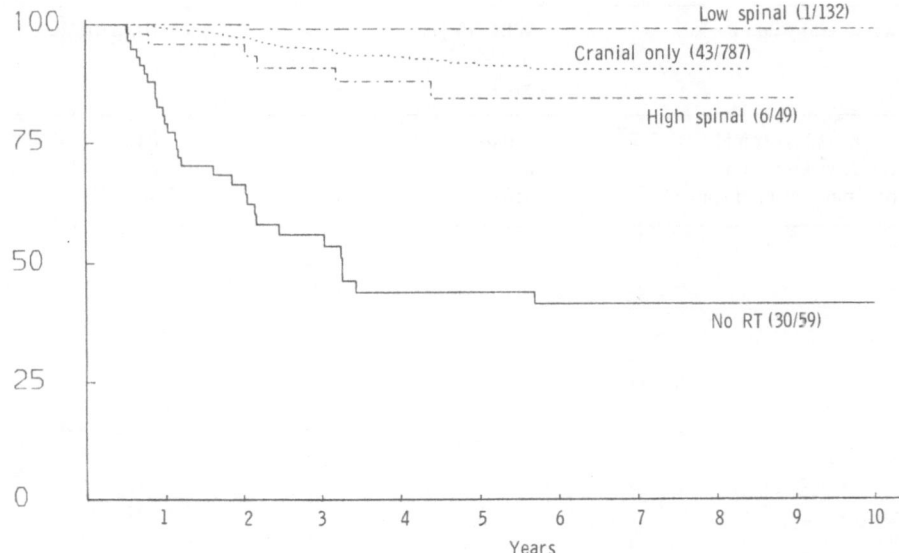

Figure 1. UKALL I–V: CNS remission duration of patients with initial leucocyte count $\leqslant 20 \times 10^9/l$, by CNS prophylactic regime. Numbers of CNS relapses (as first event) and total patients are shown for each group.

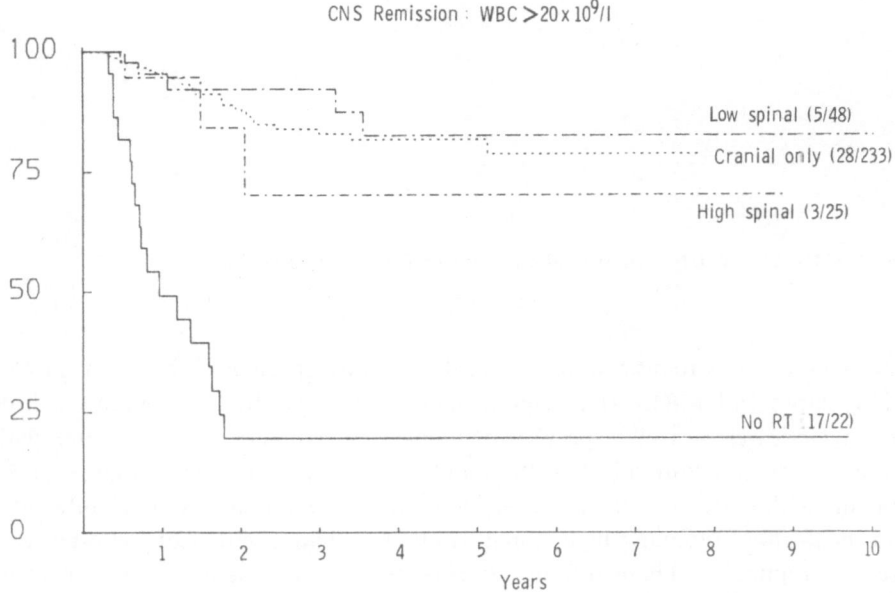

Figure 2. UKALL I–IV: CNS remission duration of patients with initial leucocyte count $> 20 \times 10^9/l$, by CNS prophylactic regime. Numbers of CNS relapses (as first event) and total patients are shown for each group.

Table 2. UKALL I–V, CNS relapse rates: significance (p) of differences between CNS prophylactic regimes.

Radiotherapy comparison	WBC($10^9/1$)		All patients
	≤20	>20	
Cranial *vs* low spinal	<0.01	n.s.	0.019
Cranial *vs* high spinal	n.s.	n.s.	n.s.
Low spinal *vs* high spinal	<0.001	n.s.	<0.002

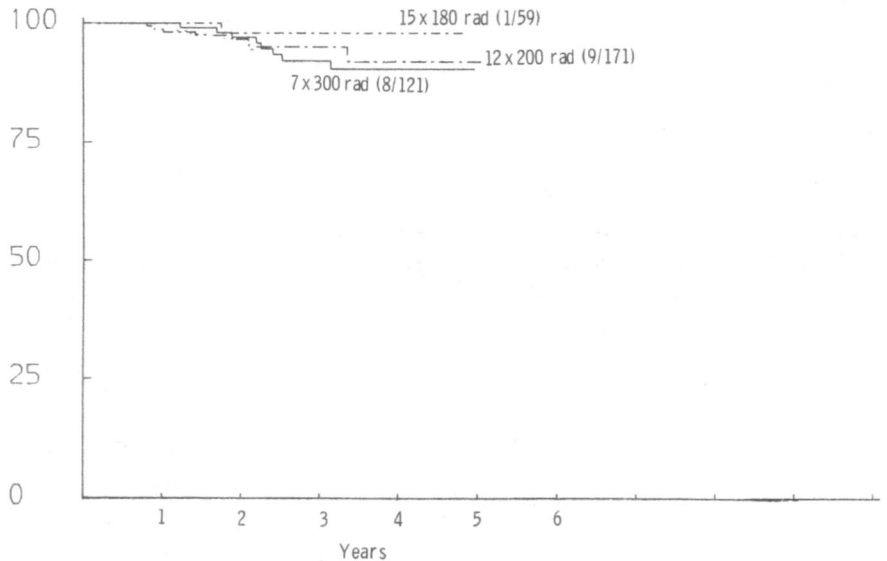

Figure 3. UKALL V: CNS remission duration by cranial radiation dosage.

first bone-marrow remission has been calculated irrespective of the occurrence of CNS relapse. In UKALL II, no significant difference was found between the three prophylactic regimes in respect to bone-marrow remission when patients with initial leucocyte counts of $20 \times 10^9/l$ and below were considered (Figure 4). In patients with higher counts, however, bone-marrow remissions were significantly shorter in those receiving high spinal irradiation than in either of the other two groups (Figure 5). These differences persisted when patients in all five trials receiving these three types of CNS prophylaxis were compared (Table 3).

In UKALL I, bone-marrow relapses were slightly, but not significantly, more frequent in patients who did not receive CNS prophylaxis than in those who did

57

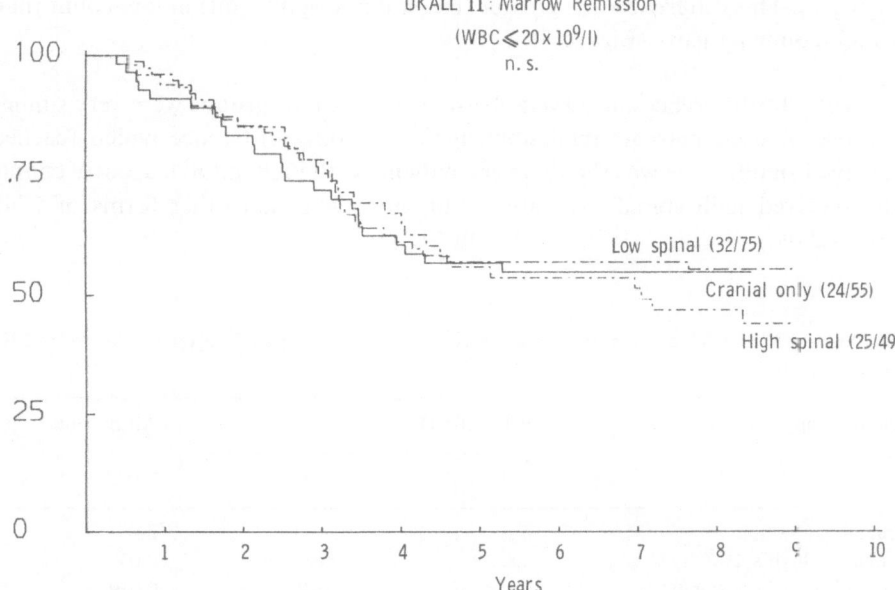

Figure 4. UKALL II: Bone-marrow remission duration of patients with initial leucocyte count ≤ 20 × 10⁹/l, by CNS prophylactic regime. Numbers of bone-marrow relapses (whether or not preceded by CNS relapse) and total patients are shown for each group.

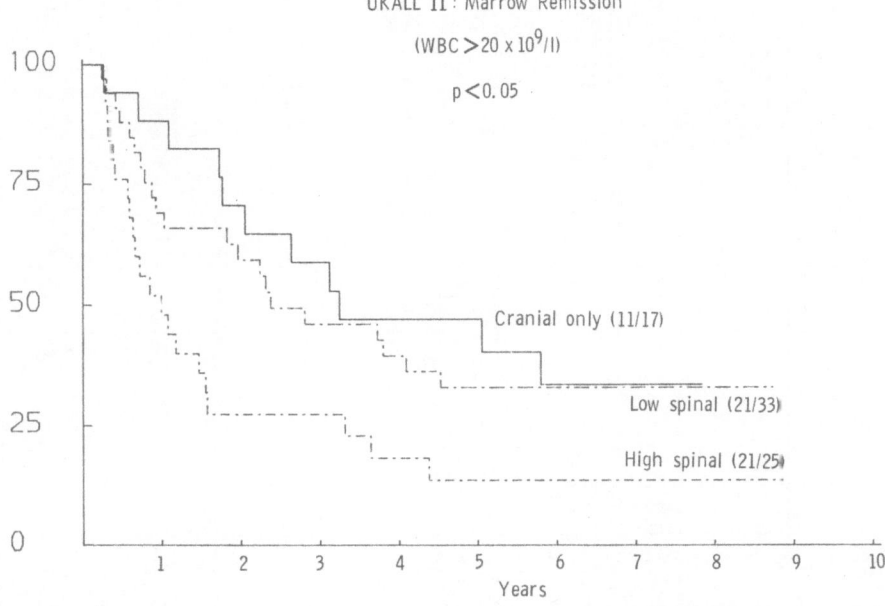

Figure 5. UKALL II: Bone-marrow remission duration of patients with initial leucocyte count > 20 × 10⁹/l, by CNS prophylactic regime. Numbers of bone-marrow relapses (whether or not preceded by CNS relapse) and total patients are shown for each group.

58

(Figure 6). This difference was greater (but still not significant) in low-count than in high-count patients (Figure 7).

Survival. The differences in survival between the various groups were very similar to those in bone-marrow remission: again, the only difference which reached statistical significance was that between patients with high initial leucocyte counts who received high spinal irradiation and those who had other forms of CNS prophylaxis.

Table 3. UKALL I–V, bone-marrow relapse rates: significance (p) of differences between CNS prophylactic regimes.

Radiotherapy comparison	WBC(10^9/1)		All patients
	$\leqslant 20$	> 20	
Cranial *vs* low spinal	n.s.	n.s.	n.s.
Cranial *vs* high spinal	n.s.	<0.01	0.06
Low spinal *vs* high spinal	n.s.	0.018	0.019

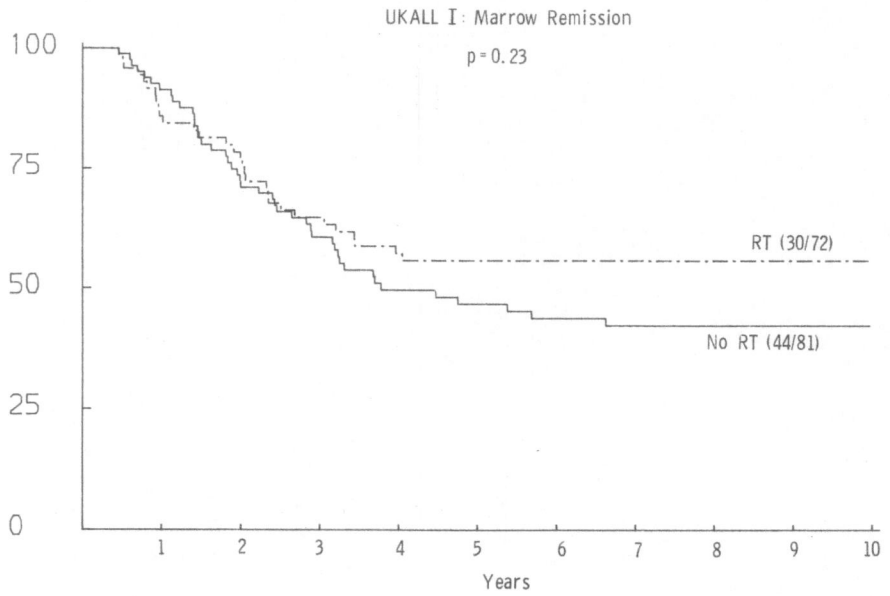

Figure 6. UKALL I: Bone-marrow remission duration of patients receiving and not receiving CNS prophylaxis.

UKALL I : Marrow Remission

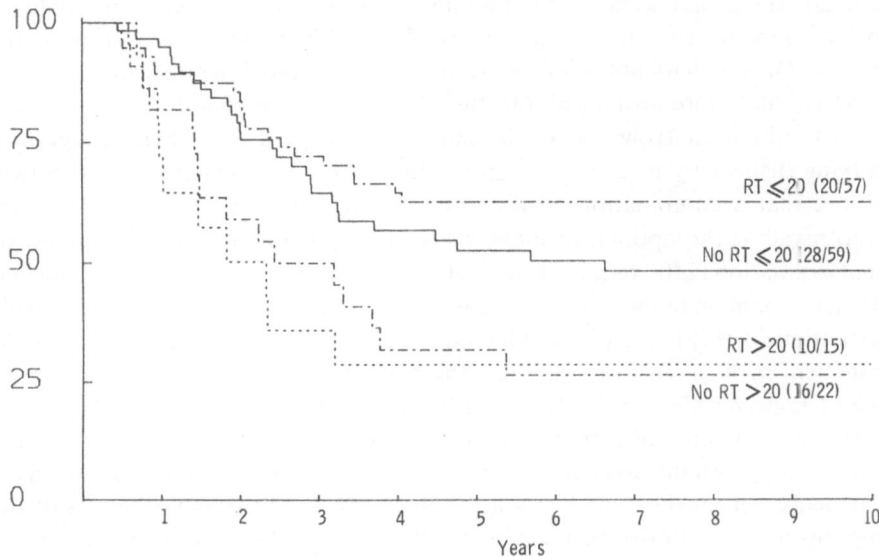

Figure 7. UKALL I: Bone-marrow remission duration of patients receiving and not receiving CNS prophylaxis, by initial leucocyte count.

Table 4. UKALL I–IV: bone marrow relapse in relation to CNS relapse.

Initial leucocyte count (× 10^9/l)	≤20		>20	
CNS prophylaxis	−	+	−	+
Total patients	59	474	22	306
CNS relapse (1st event)	30 (51)	24 (5)	17 (82)	38 (12)
Marrow relapse:				
Without CNS relapse	9 (15)	180 (38)	1 (5)	175 (57)
After CNS relapse	19 (32)	15 (3)	15 (68)	27 (9)
Total	28 (47)	195 (41)	16 (73)	202 (66)

Percentages in parentheses

Discussion

These results must be interpreted with caution, since the five trials differed with respect to induction and maintenance chemotherapy as well as CNS prophylaxis, and since some of the allocations to different treatment regimes within trials were made on a non-randomized or only partially randomized basis. Comparison of bone-marrow remission durations between individual trials, however, does not reveal any significant secular trend for either high- or low-leucocyte-count patients considered separately, and the same is true for both CNS remission duration and survival. Of the patients who received low-dose spinal irradiation, those in UKALL I had more prolonged intrathecal chemotherapy than those in UKALL II, but the bone marrow and CNS relapse rates of each were almost identical, justifying their analysis as a single group. In so far as conclusions can be drawn, they are that a combination of 1000 rad and at least five doses of intrathecal methotrexate is the optimal prophylaxis for the spinal cord, and that high-dose spinal irradiation (2400 rad) is the least effective, and may be positively deleterious in terms of bone-marrow relapse, at least for high-count patients. The most likely explanation of this latter effect, which others have also observed (7), is that the consequent myelosuppression reduces the patient's tolerance of cytotoxic drugs.

The Children's Cancer Study Group (7) has recently presented evidence that 1800 rad is as effective as 2400 rad in preventing CNS relapse, whether given to the cranium only, with intrathecal methotrexate, or to the craniospinal axis. We have no evidence yet on this point, and it is still too early to assess the results of the comparison of fractionation regimes in UKALL V, which includes a group of patients who received the intermediate total dose of 2100 rad. The most favourable regime in this trial to date, in which the smallest fractions are given over the longest period, is that which has been shown to have the greatest effect on the circulating lymphocyte count (8) but the smallest effect on pituitary function (9).

With the exception of the deleterious effect of high-dose spinal irradiation, discussed above, our findings support the conclusion of Nesbit et al (10) that the bone-marrow relapse rate in ALL is not significantly affected by CNS prophylaxis. The incidence of bone-marrow and CNS relapse in UKALL I–IV, for patients receiving or not receiving CNS prophylaxis, is summarized according to initial leucocyte count in Table IV. Although the risk of bone-marrow relapse is greater in those who relapse in the CNS than in those who never do so, this association holds whether or not CNS prophylaxis has been given. Thus the incidence of subsequent bone-marrow relapse in low-count patients who had had CNS relapse as a first event was 63% in both prophylaxis and no-prophylaxis groups (15/24 and 19/30 respectively), while the corresponding rates for high-count patients were 71% (27/38) and 88% (15/17). A tendency to relapse in the CNS is presumably determined by the same growth characteristics of leukaemic cell lines, whether or not these are reflected in the initial leucocyte count or other recognized prognostic features, as determine a tendency to relapse in the bone marrow. Bone-marrow relapse is not a direct consequence of CNS relapse, but the prevention of both provides much the surest way of eradicating the leukaemia.

Acknowledgement

We are indebted to the Medical Research Council Working Party of Leukemia in Childhood, on whose trials this report is based.

References

1. Hustu HO, Aur RJA, Verzosa MS, Simone JV, Pinkel D: Prevention of central nervous system leukemia by irradiation. Cancer 32:585–597, 1973.
2. Medical Research Council: Treatment of acute lymphoblastic leukaemia: effect of 'prophylactic' therapy against central nervous system leukaemia. Brit Med J 2:381–384, 1973.
3. Medical Research Council: Effects of varying radiation schedule, cyclophosphamide treatment, and duration of treatment in acute lymphoblastic leukaemia. Brit Med J 2:787–791, 1978.
4. Medical Research Council: The treatment of acute lymphoblastic leukaemia in childhood, UKALL III. The effects of added cytosine arabinoside and/or asparaginase, and a comparison of continuous or discontinuous mercaptopurine in regimens for standard risk ALL. Med Paed Oncol In Press, 1981.
5. Rapson NT, Cornbleet MA, Chessells JM, Bennett AJ, Hardisty RM: Immunosuppression and serious infections in children with acute lymphoblastic leukaemia: a comparison of three chemotherapy regimes. Brit J Haemat 45:41–52, 1980.
6. Peto R, Pike MC, Armitage P, Breslow NE, Cox DR, Howard SV, Mantel N, McPherson K, Peto J, Smith PG: Design and analysis of randomized clinical trials requiring prolonged observation of each patient. II. Analysis and examples. Brit J Cancer 35:1–39, 1977.
7. Nesbit ME, Sather HN, Robison LL, Ortega J, Littman PS, D'Angio GJ, Hammond GD: Presymptomatic central nervous system therapy in previously untreated childhood acute lymphoblastic leukaemia: comparison of 1800 rad and 2400 rad. Lancet 1:461–466, 1981.
8. Medical Research Council: Analysis of treatment in childhood leukaemia. IV. The critical association between dose fractionation and immunosuppression induced by cranial irradiation. Cancer 41:108–11, 1978.
9. Shalet SM, Beardwell CG, Morris Jones PH, Pearson D: Growth hormone deficiency after treatment of acute leukaemia in children. Arch Dis Childh 51:489–493, 1976.
10. Nesbit ME, D'Angio GJ, Sather HN, Robison LL, Ortega J, Donaldson M, Hammond GD: Effect of isolated central nervous system leukaemia on bone marrow remission and survival in childhood acute lymphoblastic leukaemia. Lancet 1: 1386–1389, 1981.

8. The Norwegian Methotrexate Study in Childhood Acute Lymphocytic Leukemia

PJ MOE, M SEIP, PH FINNE, and S KOLMANNSKOG

The ability to cure children with leukemia has focused attention on the long term sequelae of therapy. A number of studies, including those presented elsewhere in this book, have indicated the potential adverse effects of the combination of cranial irradiation and intrathecal methotrexate. Therefore we have tried to avoid prophylactic cranial irradiation in our treatment protocol.

Intermediate dose methotrexate (IDM) with leucovorin rescue therapy as primary 'sanctuary' treatment following induction therapy was introduced by Freeman and his colleagues (1, 2). A similar program using IDM was started in Norway in August 1975 (3). The major differences being that CNS prophylaxis with weekly intrathecal methotrexate (MTX) instillation was begun at the start of antileukemic therapy instead of after the induction period, and that 8 doses were given intrathecally instead of 6 doses (Figure 1.). Our experience with this protocol was published earlier (3, 4, 5). In the beginning of 1980 it was decided to increase the dose of intravenous MTX from 0.5 to 4–$8 \, g/m^2$ (HDM) per 24 hours in cases with marked leukocytosis (WBC above $50 \times 10^9/l$).

No prophylactic irradiation was used in this study.

Material and methods

A survey of the material is presented in Tables 1 and 2. In August-December 1975 only a few departments of pediatrics were using the IDM protocol, while since early in 1976 all pediatric departments in Norway treating children with leukemia have participated.

A total of 14 patients diagnosed before 1976 received IDM courses while they were in complete primary remission. Six of these are not included in the statistical analysis because they received IDM courses while they were in a later phase of treatment and therefore do not fit into the protocol. Four of the 6 cases are still off therapy and in continuous complete remission (CCR). The same treatment protocol was originally planned for two additional cases in 1975. However, a 10-month-old female with an initial WBC of $700 \times 10^9/l$ received one course of MTX while she was in incomplete remission and a $3\frac{1}{2}$ year old male died of infection without achieving remission.

R. Mastrangelo, D.G. Poplack, R. Riccardi (eds), Central Nervous System Leukemia. ISBN 978-94-009-6710-6.
© 1983 Martinus Nijhoff Publishers, Boston.

Altogether 141 cases have been diagnosed as acute lymphoblastic leukemia (ALL) in Norway in children under 15 years old in the 5-year period 1976–1980, (Table 1). One hundred and eighteen of them received the IDM protocol while they were in complete remission and 6 in the increased risk (IR) group received the protocol using HDM instead of IDM.

The total material thus consists of 132 cases (51 girls and 81 boys) from 1975–1980 receiving IDM or HDM (6 cases) while they were in their complete remission, and a mixed group of 19 cases (8 boys and 11 girls) who for various reasons did not receive IDM/HDM while they were in complete remission (Table 2). Eight (5.3%) of the total 151 cases of ALL did not achieve remission (Tables 1 and 2).

Only five of the total 82 cases diagnosed as childhood ALL in Norway during the the 3-year period 1978–1980 did not receive IDM/HDM while they were in complete remission. Three of them died early in the induction phase, one was treated in a department of internal medicine not using our protocol – she relapsed after

Table 1. Shows a survey of the material, total 151 cases.

Diagnosis (year)	Patients receiving IDM or HDM in complete remission			Other cases of ALL			All cases
	SR	IR	Total	SR	IR	Total	
1975	6	2	8	1	1	2	(10)
1976	15	9	24	5	2	7	31
1977	15	8	23	3	2	5	28
1978	13	6	19	0	1	1	20
1979	13	11	24	1	2	3	27
1980	19	15	34	1	0	1	35
Total	81	51	132	11	8	19	151

Table 2. A survey of the 19 cases not receiving IDM in CR.

Diagnosis (year)	Not achieving complete remission	Died early in remiss.	Treated with other protoc.	No treatment Downs syndrome
1975	2	0	–	–
1976	2	2	3	0
1977	1	2	1	1
1978	1	0	0	0
1979	1	0	2	0
1980	1	0	0	0
Total	8 (5.3%)	4 (2.6%)	6 (4.0%)	1

about $\frac{1}{2}$ year – and the fifth child is still in remission. She developed convulsions following vincristine combined with intrathecal MTX, and she therefore received a different protocol.

The children have been separated into standard risk (SR) and increased risk (IR) patients. We defined increased risk as a WBC over $30 \times 10^9/l$ and/or age less than 2 years or greater than 10 years at diagnosis. CNS leukemia at the time of diagnosis (present in 2 of 151 cases) and mediastinal mass (2 cases) were also considered as IR factors. As shown in Table 1 there were 81 SR and 51 IR patients in the group receiving MTX infusions and 11 SR and 8 IR patients in the mixed group.

The mixed group not included in the calculation of life tables (Table 2) consisted of 8 patients (5.3%) not achieving complete remission, 4 patients dying of early infection while in complete remission, 6 patients treated with other protocols, and one patient with Down's syndrome not given antileukemic treatment. In addition there have been 3 patients with unclassified leukemia in children in Norway in 1976–1980. Two of them died early, before the diagnostic work-up was completed, and the parents refused therapy in a child with leukemia and Down's syndrome.

Statistical analysis of disease-free period and survival has been performed using the Kaplan-Meier method for calculating and projecting curves. Only the first 95 children receiving IDM while they were in their first remission are included in the calculation of life tables. All of them had been followed for at least 18 months. The observation time for the other children receiving methotrexate infusions while in complete remission is shorter than 18 months. The disease-free survival curves, however, are practically identical whether the 37 patients receiving IDM/HDM after January 1980 are included or not. The induction protocol consisted of vincristine plus dexamethasone or prednisone (since January 1978), followed by L-asparaginase for 10 days. In 46 cases the protocol did not include L-asparaginase. In 27 of these 46 cases 6-mercaptopurine was used after two weeks in the induction phase in addition to the combination of vincristine and steroids. Furthermore, a combination of cytosine arabinoside, adriamycin and cyclophosphamide was used instead of L-asparaginase in one department in 14 IR patients.

After complete remission had been achieved, and after the use of L-asparaginase or the above mentioned combination induction, three infusions of MTX were administered intravenously at 3 weekly intervals. One third of the IDM dose was given as a bolus and the remaining 2/3 in a 24 hour infusion. Twenty-four hours following the completion of the infusion of MTX, a single dose of leucovorin (citrovorum factor), $12\,mg/m^2$, was given. Since October 1976, two doses of leucovorin have been used, 24 and 36 hours following the infusion, respectively.

The maintenance phase consisted of daily oral 6 mercaptopurine and weekly oral MTX, and reinforcements with steroids and vincristine (Figure 1).

In the 6 cases in IR-group 4–$6\,g/m^2$ MTX was used in 24 hour infusions, $1/10^{th}$

66

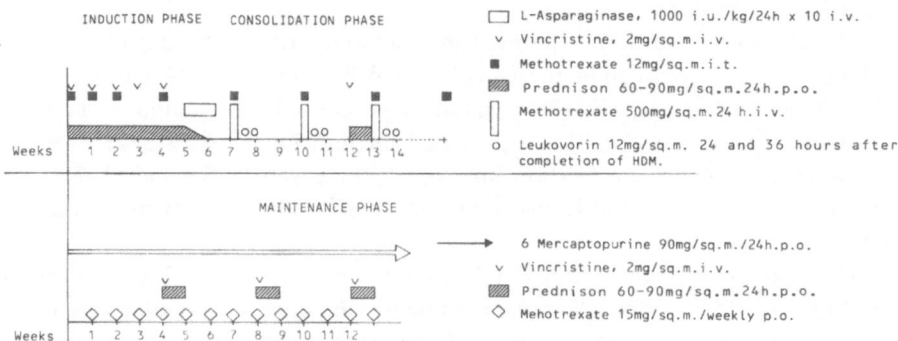

Treatment protocol for children with ALL.

Figure 1. IDM-treatment protocol for children with ALL.

of the dose was given as a bolus, and 16 doses of citrovorum factor were given instead of 2 due to the higher dose of MTX. Treatment has been discontinued after 2 to 3 years of CCR. Before discontinuation of therapy all patients had normal bone marrow and spinal fluid.

Results

All the 132 children survived the IDM/HDM therapy, but serious reactions occurred in several cases (Table 3). The dose had to be reduced in 12 (8%) cases due to previous adverse reactions. The most severe reactions were seen before two doses of leucovorin were introduced in the IDM protocol (4).

Life table of CCR for the first 95 patients and for the 62 cases in SR and 33 IR patients are shown in Figure 2. The disease-free survival curves are practically

Table 3. Untoward reactions to IDM in 34 out of 132 cases.

Untoward reactions to IDM	No. of cases
Pancytopenia + sepsis (?) + stomatitis	2
Convulsions following intrathecal MTX + IDM	1
Cytomegal ovirus infection + stomatitis	1
Skin reactions (Stevens-Johnson's syndrome in 2) + stomatitis	9
Stomatitis in other cases	20
Pharyngitis	1
Total (out of 132 cases)	34

identical whether the 37 cases receiving IDM/HDM after January 1980 are included or not.

Survival curves for 95 cases only are shown in Figure 3. A total of 18 (19%) had died within June 1981. The deaths of 5 cases in CCR in 1976–77 markedly influence both the disease-free survival and the survival curve for the SR group, as all 5 cases belonged to that group. No child has died during the last 4 years in CCR.

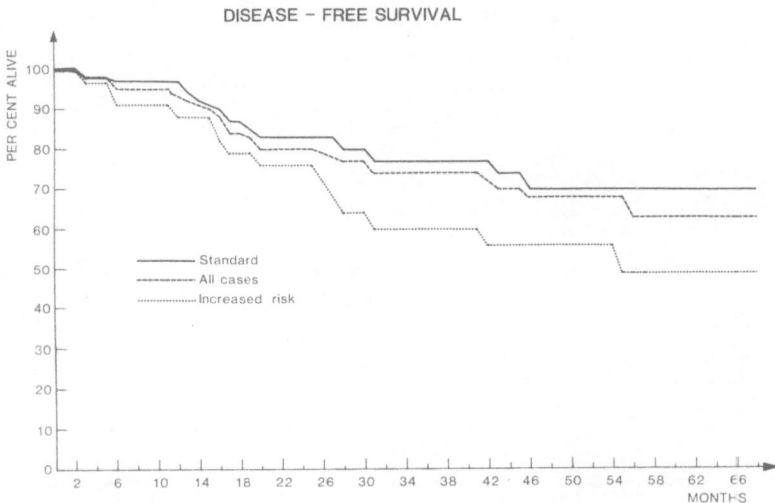

Figure 2. Length of CCR in 95 children with ALL in Norway treated with IDM.

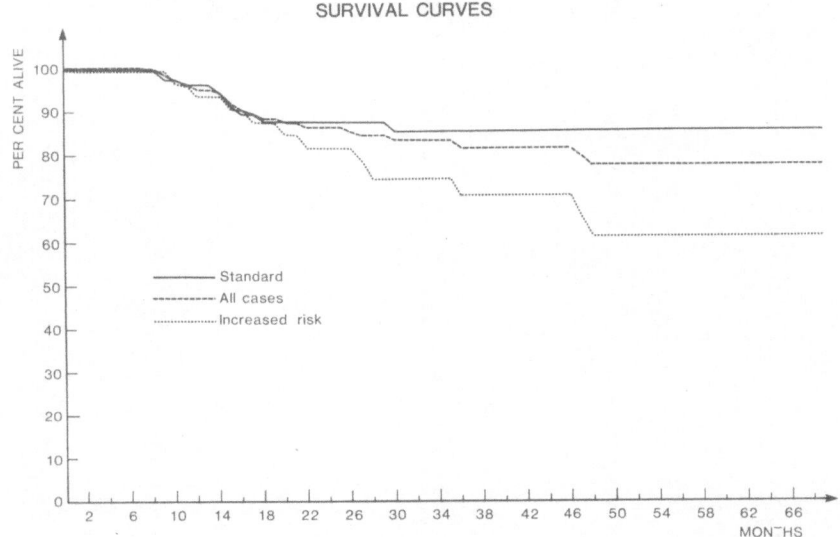

Figure 3. Survival curves in the 95 children with ALL in Norway treated with IDM.

68

The first 95 children receiving IDM/HDM in Norway have been followed for 18–69 months, with a median of 45 months. The relapse rate has been 23/95 (24%) as of June 1981 with the CNS as the initial site of relapse 7 (7.3%). Figure 4 shows the disease-free survival for primary isolated CNS-relapse.

In addition there were 4 cases of combined systemic and CNS-relapse. Figure 5 shows the disease-free survival for both primary CNS and combined systemic and CNS-relapses for the first 95 cases with a follow-up of at least 18 months.

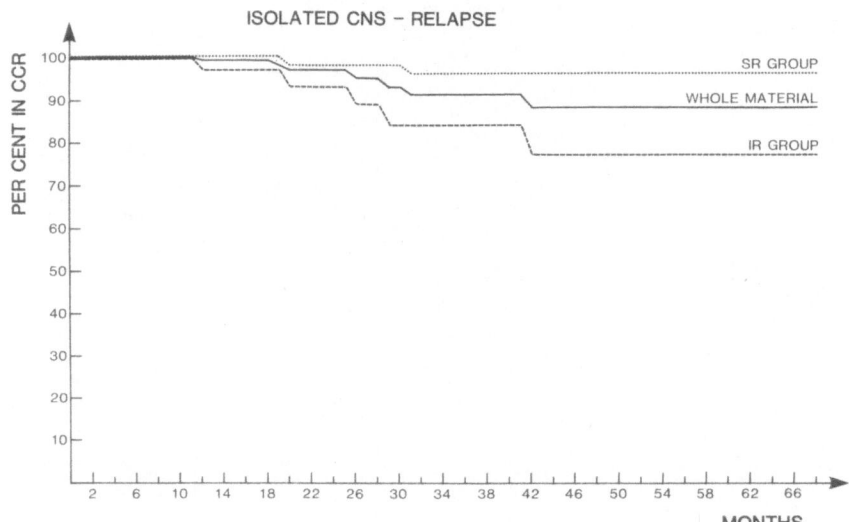

Figure 5. Disease free survival for both primary CNS and combined systemic and CNS-relapse.

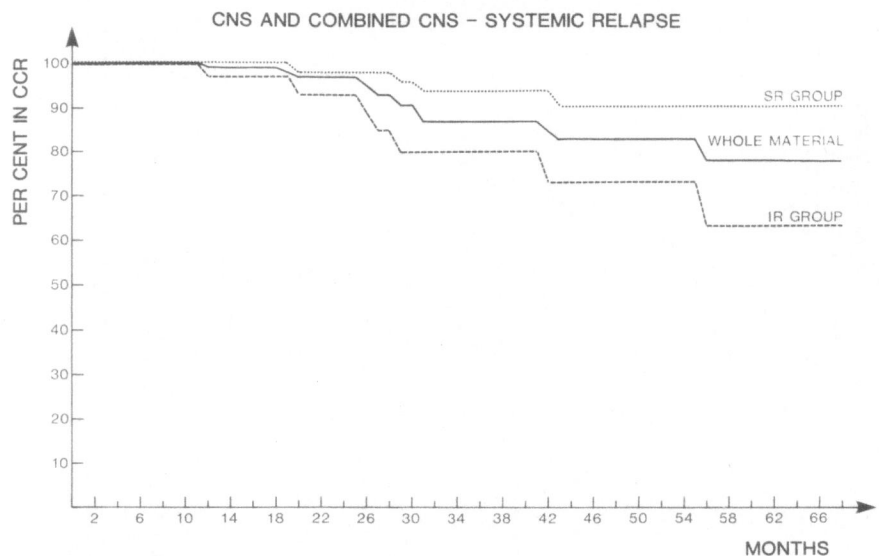

Figure 4. Disease free survival for primary CNS-relapse.

Discussion

The first 95 cases receiving IDM have been followed for 18–69 months with a median of 45 months. The over all relapse rate has been 24%, with the CNS as initial isolated site of relapse in 7.3%. In addition there were 4 combined systemic and CNS-relapses. This study thus indicates an efficacy of 8 doses of Methotrexate intrathecally combined with IDM in preventing meningeal leukemia in patients with ALL, comparable with the results obtained with cranial irradiation combined with IT MTX (6, 7). There were, however, a total of 11 cases with CNS involvement among the 23 relapses.

Not a single case of gonadal involvement and only one case of other sanctuary relapse (a tumor in the subcutaneous tissue), have been diagnosed in our study so far. Gonadal and other sanctuaries are probably the main sources of systemic relapse in ALL.

It seems that successful cessation of therapy will take place in 70–75% of all cases who received IDM while in sustained remission or in 60–65% of the total material. The relapse rate after cessation of therapy, approximately 12%, is relatively low. The follow-up after cessation, however, still is short in many of the cases. Further follow-up is indicated in order to evaluate the ultimate long-term efficacy of our treatment protocol.

References

1. Freeman AI, Wang JJ, Sinks LF: High dose methotrexate in acute lymphocytic leukemia (ALL) Abstract 16th International Congress of Hematology, Kyote, September 1976.
2. Wang JJ, Freeman AI, Sinks LF: Treatment of acute lymphocytic leukemia by high dose intravenous methotrexate. Cancer Res 36:1441–1444, 1980.
3. Moe PJ, Seip M: High dose methotrexate in acute lympholytic leukemia in children. Acta Paediatr Scand 67:265–268, 1978.
4. Moe PJ, Seip M, Finne PH: Intermediate dose of methotrexate in childhood leukemia in Norway. Acta Paediatr Scand 70:73–79, 1981.
5. Moe PJ, Seip M, Finne PH: Intermediate dose of methotrexate (IDM) in childhood acute lymphocytic leukemia in Norway. Follow up on a national treatment protocol. Exerpta Medica. In press.
6. Riehm H, Gadner H, Welte K: Die West-Berliner Studie zur Behandlung der Akute Lymphatischen Leukemiäe des Kindes-Erfahrungsbericht nach 6 Jahren. Klin Pädiatr 189:89–102, 1977.
7. Simone JV et al: Combined modality therapy of acute lymphocytic leukemia. Cancer 35:25–35, 1975.

9. Therapy Related Central Nervous System Diseases in Children with Acute Lymphocytic Leukemia

R.A. PRICE

Introduction

Before 1950 the prognosis for children with acute lymphocytic leukemia was uniformly poor. Despite therapy that included blood transfusion and occasionally irradiation to enlarged viscera and mediastinal masses, the majority of children who developed this disease died during the first six months following diagnosis, and rarely did a child survive beyond nine months (1). Farber's success. reported in 1948, in achieving temporary remissions in five children with leukemia by using the folic acid antagonist 4-aminopteroyl-glutamic acid led to the development of more potent anti-leukemic drugs capable of prolonging these initial remissions (2). These early achievements demonstrated that extracranial leukemia could be controlled by chemotherapy; however, meningeal leukemia proved to be more resistant. Cranial radiation of 1500 rads or less provided temporary gains and similar attempts to eradicate leukemic cells from the central nervous system (CNS) by intrathecal injection of drugs were equally unsuccessful (3–7). Meningeal leukemia occurring during remission was usually followed by hematological relapse, leaving little chance for cure. Thus CNS leukemia was identified as one of the main obstacles to the successful treatment of acute leukemia in children.

Effective control of meningeal leukemia was obtained by increasing the dose of radiation. By using a dose of 2000–2400 rads to the cranium and combining this with more intensive chemotherapy, Pinkel and his associates developed treatment programs which led to five year complete remissions in over 40% of children with acute lymphocytic leukemia (ALL) (8–10).

Although the signs and symptoms of meningeal leukemia (11) were clearly identified before 1970, the trend to more intensive CNS therapy was soon accompanied by reports of unusual neurological abnormalities that could not be accounted for on the basis of meningeal leukemia alone (12–25). Over the past decade three distinctive neurological complications of current treatment methods for acute lymphocytic leukemia have been recognized: subacute leukoencephalopathy, mineralizing microangiopathy and subacute necrotizing leukomyelopathy. This paper reviews pathological characteristics, selected clinical features and pathogenesis in these three diseases.

R. Mastrangelo, D.G. Poplack, R. Riccardi (eds), Central Nervous System Leukemia. ISBN 978-94-009-6710-6.
© *1983 Martinus Nijhoff Publishers, Boston.*

Subacute leukoencephalopathy

This complication of therapy in children and young adults treated for acute lymphocytic leukemia affects the white matter of the brain. Grey matter is characteristically spared. The early histopathologic characteristics consist of areas of reactive astrocytosis, necrosis of myelin sheaths and neuronal processes, and macrophages (Figure 1). As the process continues, necrotic foci become confluent and extensive white matter degeneration and cavitation occurs (Figure 2). The occasional mineralized cellular debris seen in the lesions should not be confused with the vascular degeneration and dystrophic calcification of mineralizing microangiopathy, which is found in CNS grey matter.

The clinical features of this complication of therapy may become apparent as early as four to five months following cranial radiation. These features include focal seizures, lethargy, ataxia, slurred speech, spasticity, dysphasia, confusion, and terminally the patients become decerebrate and comatose. The electro-encephalogram (EEG) is abnormal (24).

Children who develop leukoencephalopathy have typically received cranial irradiation, intrathecal methotrexate (IT MTX), and intravenous methotrexate (IV MTX) treatments. Patients at highest risk to develop this disease are those who receive cranial irradiation of 2000–2400 rads and IT MTX followed by IV

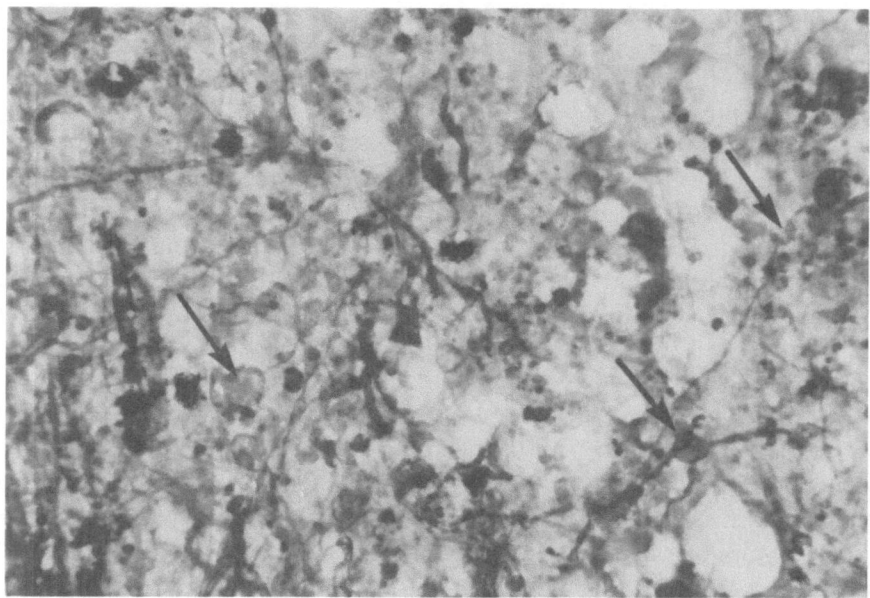

Figure 1. Marked central white matter necrosis consisting of pyknotic, karyorrhectic neuroglial debris and myelin-sheath disintegration. Note focal swellings of myelin sheaths (arrows). (Luxol-fast blue with H&E counterstain. × 538). Courtesy of Cancer (24).

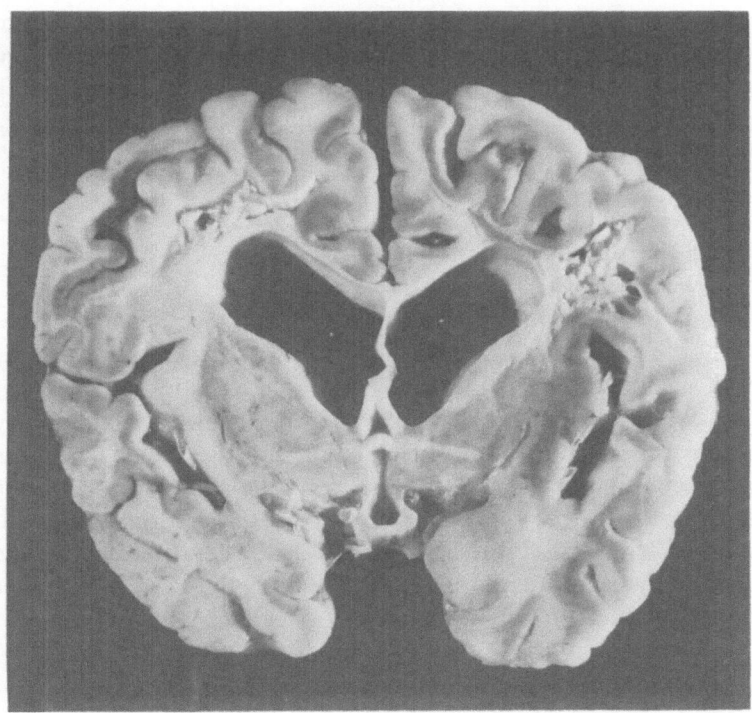

Figure 2. Coronal section of brain demonstrating principal features of advanced leukoencephalopathy. Note enlarged lateral ventricles and necrotic cystic frontal lobe white matter. Courtesy of Martinus Nijhoff Publishers (30).

MTX in weekly doses of $50 \, mg/m^2$. In one clinical trial, 50% of children receiving this treatment developed leukoencephalopathy (26). A second group at considerably lower risk consists of children who receive similar radiation doses, and IT MTX, and IV MTX at doses of $20 \, mg/m^2$, then develop CNS and bone marrow relapses necessitating additional chemotherapy and occasionally second treatments of cranial irradiation. Another group in which leukoencephalopathy may develop are those patients receiving cranial irradiation of 3500 rads or more and chemotherapy for clinically evident meningeal leukemia (18). This complication of therapy has not yet been reported in children who received irradiation, IT MTX and oral methotrexate maintenance therapy, regardless of the number of CNS and hematological relapses suffered during the course of their disease.

Although the precise relationship of radiation and chemotherapy to the development of leukoencephalopathy has been difficult to define, the well-characterized effects of radiation on the microvasculature provide a basis for the following hypothesis: radiation treatment alters the permeability of the blood-brain-barrier (BBB) which then allows methotrexate to diffuse into the brain and

74

cause necrosis of white matter. Although it has long been known from animal studies that radiation can render the BBB more permeable (27), only recently has this been shown for methotrexate (28). This drug was recovered from the brains of mice treated with 2000 rads of cranial irradiation given in a single dose, but not from animals pretreated with lower doses or non-irradiated controls (28).

Mineralizing microangiopathy

The hallmark of mineralizing microangiopathy is the presence of focal CNS calcifications. This disease is a noninflammatory, degenerative and mineralizing disorder of small vessels accompanied by dystrophic calcification of adjacent brain tissue (25). Whereas leukoencephalopathy affects CNS white matter, mineralizing microangiopathy is confined to grey matter. The disease usually begins in vessels of the putamen (Figure 3), and later appears in arterial border zone regions of the cerebral cortex. In severe cases large areas of cerebral cortex are involved and eventually the cerebellar cortex becomes affected. The diagnosis of mineralizing microangiopathy can be easily made on the basis of striking computed tomographic (CT) findings (Figure 4).

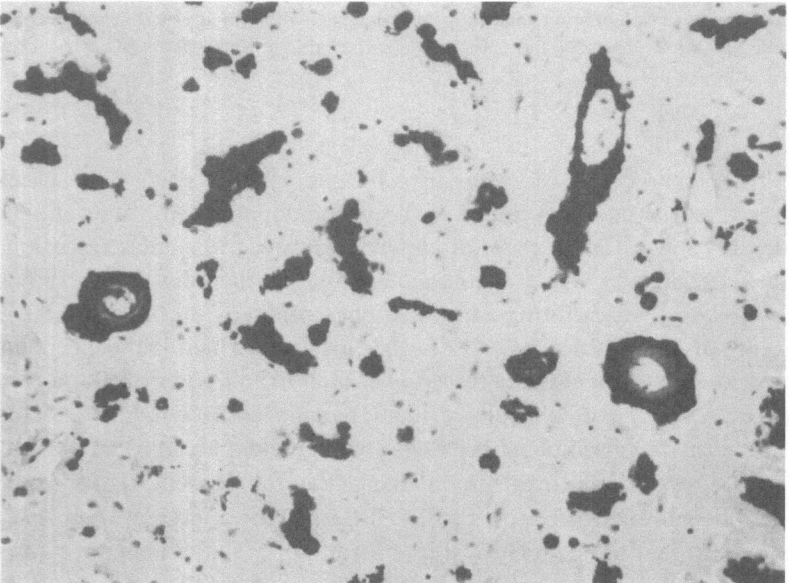

Figure 3. Mineralizing microangiopathy in putamen nucleus. Lumens of most smaller vessels are occluded by precipitated mineralized material. Although larger vessels have patent lumens, their walls contain conspicuous amounts of mineralized debris (H & E, × 136). Courtesy of Cancer (25).

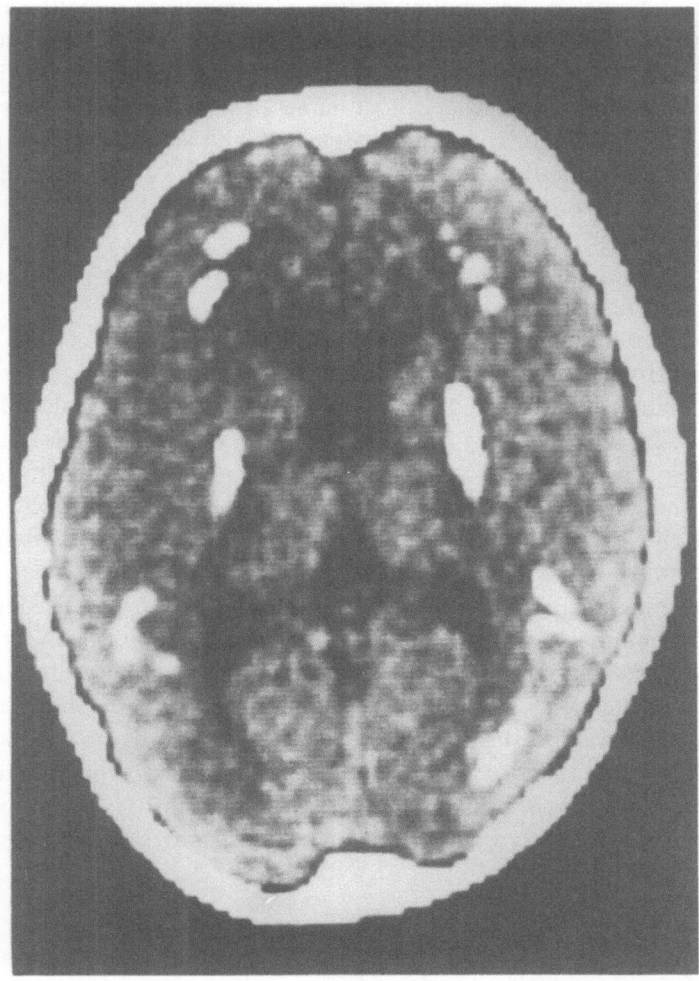

Figure 4. Characteristic computed tomographic features of mineralizing microangiopathy. Calcifications are present in putamen nuclei and in cerebral cortex border zones between anterior, middle and posterior cerebral arteries.

Neurological abnormalities described in patients with these CNS calcifications include seizures, poor muscular control, ataxia, memory deficits and behavioral disorders. The EEG is also abnormal. The relationship of these clinical observations to the progression of the histologic changes of mineralizing microangiopathy and the calcifications that characterize this disease is still to be clarified.

Several variables associated with the development of mineralizing micro-angiopathy have been identified. Two factors are the age of the patient at the time of cranial irradiation and the amount of time elapsing after radiation treatment. Children 10 years old or younger at time of radiotherapy are more susceptible than adolescents, and children younger than 6 years are especially vulnerable. Radiologic and histologic evidence of mineralizing microangiopathy usually becomes apparent nine or ten months after cranial irradiation (23, 25). A third factor which appears to influence the development of mineralizing microangiopathy is chemotherapy. One study demonstrated that 30% of the most vulnerable children receiving high doses of IV MTX and cytosine arabinoside developed cerebral calcifications during their initial complete clinical remission following induction therapy and radiotherapy (23).

Other factors also may be important in the development of this lesion. A significant increase in the number of cases of mineralizing microangiopathy was found in children who received additional therapy for meningeal and hematological relapses. Since the study was retrospective, it was not possible to determine whether the increased frequency of vascular disease was related to additional therapy, meningeal leukemia, or a combination of the two (25). However, there is little convincing evidence to indicate that meningeal leukemia is a primary cause of this mineralizing vascular disease.

Although mineralizing microangiopathy is found in children with leukemia who have received cranial radiation and systemic chemotherapy, the exact determinants of its frequency and outcome are not yet known. Many other questions remain unanswered. Why are the arterial border zones of the cerebral vasculature particularly vulnerable? If the disease appears in the basal ganglia, will it inevitably progress to affect cerebral and cerebellar cortex? What determines the rate of this process? And finally, what is the incidence of this disease in treated children who survive with a complete clinical remission?

Subacute necrotizing leukomyelopathy

During routine examinations of the CNS of children who died with ALL, an unsuspected spinal cord lesion was found. This lesion was not confined to patients who had received spinal irradiation. Sixty-five spinal cords were examined and twenty had this distinctive alteration called subacute necrotizing leukomyelopathy (Price, unpublished data).

The principal histopathologic characteristics of this lesion are myelin and axonal necrosis, macrophage infiltration, and the presence of sudanophilic positive material indicative of myelin degradation. Gliosis, though not a prominent feature, was present in more severely affected cases. Inflammation and vascular lesions were not present. Meningeal leukemia was present rarely. The mildest form of leukomyelopathy consisted of focal areas of myelin necrosis and macrophage infiltration in either the lateral or posterior columns, or both, of the thoracic spinal cord. In more advanced cases the posterior and lateral column necrosis extended to the lower thoracic and lumbar cord caudally, and rostrally as high as the lower cervical cord. In the most severe form, the disease was indistinguishable from subacute combined degeneration of cobalamine deficiency (Figure 5).

The relationship of subacute necrotizing leukomyelopathy to seventeen clinical and pathological features are shown in Table 1. The five variables considered significant were a) peripheral white blood count (WBC) at diagnosis, b) risk group characteristics, c) response to induction therapy, d) survival time, and e) megaloblastic anemia. The first four features – WBC, risk characteristics, induction response, and survival time – were interdependent. Megaloblastic anemia, though strongly associated with spinal cord disease, was not related to the first four variables. Logistic regression analysis of these five variables identified initial WBC, survival time, and megaloblastic anemia as the features most useful in identifying patients with subacute necrotizing leukomyelopathy at autopsy. The association between leukomyelopathy and patients with lower WBC at diagnosis is not a pathogenetic association. Rather, this statistical relationship reflects these patients' favorable response to induction therapy and hence longer survival time. Eighty-four percent of all cases of spinal cord disease occurred in children who had survived two years or more following diagnosis of leukemia. Although serum folate levels were not analyzed in these patients, we propose that the principal

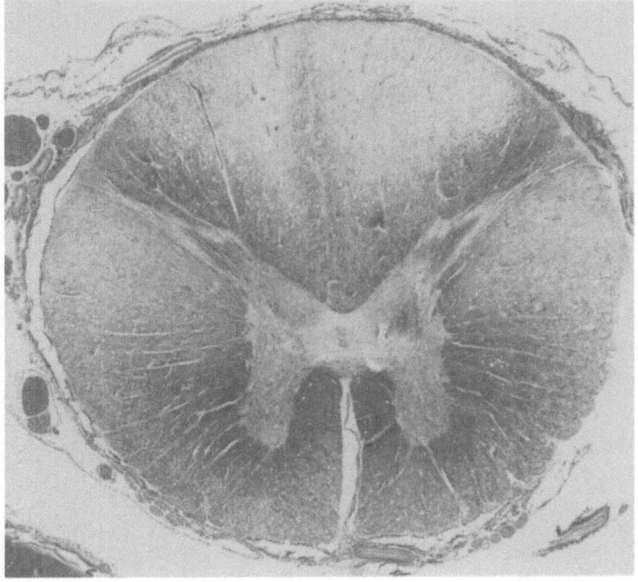

Figure 5. Cross section of midthoracic spinal cord from patient with subacute necrotizing leuko-myelopathy. The distribution of the lesions of this disease are remarkably similar to the spinal cord changes of cobalamine deficiency. (Luxol-fast blue with H & E counterstain, × 7).

Table 1. Relationship of clinical and pathological features to subacute necrotizing leukomyelopathy.

Feature	No. of patient	Leukomyelopathy		p value*
		Yes	No	
Sex				
Male	38	10	28	0.419
Female	27	10	17	
Race				
White	53	15	38	
Other	12	5	7	0.490
Age at diagnosis (years)				
<5	24	7	17	
5–14	22	7	15	0.977
≥15	19	6	13	
WBC × 10³ at diagnosis				
<10	21	9	12	
10–99	32	11	21	*0.031*
≥100	12	0	12	
CNS leukemia at diagnosis				
Yes	3	1	2	
No	62	20	45	1.000
Mediastinal mass at diagnosis				
Yes	8	1	7	
No	57	19	38	0.417
E-Rosette				
+	6	0	6	
−	41	11	30	0.312
Response to induction				
CR	55	20	35	
No CR	10	0	10	*0.025*
Spinal cord irradiation				
Yes	7	3	4	
No	38	17	41	0.667
Risk group				
Standard	50	19	31	*0.026*
High	15	1	14	
No. of bone marrow relapses				
<2	14	3	14	
2	16	8	16	0.268
≥3	25	9	25	
No. of CNS relapses				
0	34	13	21	
1	16	5	11	0.878
≥2	5	2	3	

Table 1. Continued.

Feature	No. of patient	Leukomyelopathy		p value*
		Yes	No	
No. times megaloblastic anemia				
0	29	4	25	
1	6	2	4	*0.017*
≥2	30	14	16	
Age at death (years)				
<8	17	4	13	
8–17	31	10	21	0.736
≥18	17	6	11	
Survival (years)				
<2	32	3	29	
2–5	25	13	12	*0.001*
≥6	8	4	4	
Mineralizing micro- angiopathy				
Yes	6	2	4	
No	59	18	41	1.000
Leukoencephalopathy				
Yes	4	1	3	
No	61	19	42	1.000

Abbreviations: CR, complete remission.
* Determined by either x^2 analysis of Fisher's exact test.
p Values in italics are considered significant.

cause of subacute necrotizing leukomyelopathy is a folate deficiency secondary to prolonged methotrexate treatment. To what extent these changes are reversible in the early stages, as is the case with treated subacute combined degeneration of vitamin B_{12}, is not yet known.

Since folate deficiency is known to cause megaloblastic anemia and myelopathy (29), studies of the etiology of subacute necrotizing leukomyelopathy must consider the role of the antifolate metabolite methotrexate in the development of this CNS disease. Analysis of autopsy and treatment records in this group of leukemic patients disclosed some interesting relationships between methotrexate therapy and leukomyelopathy. Fifty percent of the children who received a cumulative dose of 1,000 mgm of methotrexate or more had myelopathy at autopsy, in contrast to a prevalence of only 17% in those receiving less than 1,000 mg. A similar relationship in the group existed between IT MTX and myelopathy. Seventy-five percent of the children who had received a cumulative dose of 200 mgm or more intrathecally had evidence of white matter necrosis in their spinal cords at autopsy.

Summary

Our understanding of the CNS complications of childhood leukemia has evolved slowly. Furthermore, the pathology of these disorders has changed remarkably since the introduction of chemotherapy and CNS radiation. In untreated patients the principal complications were meningeal leukemia, hemorrhage, and infection. Currently neurotoxic effects related to radiation and chemotherapy attract greater attention than the lesions traditionally associated with meningeal leukemia.

This paper reviews the histopathologic features, selected clinical manifestations, and pathogenesis of three therapy-related CNS diseases: 1) subacute leuko-encephalopathy, a disease caused by combination of radiation followed by IV MTX treatments; 2) mineralizing microangiopathy, a disease of small vessels exposed to radiation in which chemotherapy plays a yet unexplained role; and 3) subacute necrotizing leukomyelopathy, a degenerative disease of the spinal cord in which the principal cause may be a drug-induced folate deficiency secondary to long term methotrexate therapy.

Only careful prospective studies can determine the consequences and incidence of these three complications. Information obtained from cranial CT scans, neurological and psychological examinations, and analysis of radiotherapy and chemotherapy will eventually lead to a greater understanding of the risks of current modes of therapy for childhood leukemia.

References

1. Cooke JV: Acute leukemia in children. JAMA 101:432–435, 1933.
2. Farber S, Diamond LK, Mercer RD *et al*: Temporary remissions in acute leukemia in children produced by folic acid antagonist, 4-aminopteroyl-glutamic acid (aminopterin). N Engl J Med 238:787–793, 1948.
3. Whiteside JA, Philips FS, Dargeon HW, Burchenal JH: Intrathecal amethopterin in neurological manifestations of leukemia. Arch Intern Med 101:279–285, 1958.
4. Hardisty RM, Norman PM: Meningeal leukemia. Arch Dis Child 42:441–447, 1967.
5. D'Angio GJ, Evans AE, Mitus A: Roentgen therapy of certain complications of acute leukemia in childhood. Am J Roentgenol 82:541–553, 1959.
6. Sullivan MP: Leukemia infiltration of meninges and spinal nerve roots. Pediatrics 32:63–72, 1963.
7. Sullivan MP, Vietti TJ, Fernbach DJ *et al*: Clinical investigations in the treatment of meningeal leukemia; radiation therapy regimens vs. conventional intrathecal methotrexate. Blood 34: 301–319, 1969.
8. Pinkel D, simone J, Hustu HO, Verzosa MS: Nine year's experience with 'Total Therapy' of childhood acute lymphocytic leukemia. Pediatrics 50:246–251, 1972.
9. Aur RJA, Simone JV, Hustu HO, Verzosa MS: A comparative study of central nervous system irradiation and intensive chemotherapy early in remission of childhood acute lymphocytic leukemia. Cancer 29:381–391, 1972.
0. Hustu HO, Aur RJA, Verzosa MS *et al*: Prevention of central nervous system leukemia by irradiation. Cancer 32:585–597, 1973.
. Hyman CB, Bogle JM, Burbaker CA *et al*: Central nervous system involvement by leukemia in

children. I. Relationship to systemic leukemia and description of clinical and laboratory manifestations. Blood 25:1–12, 1965.

12. Kay HEM, Knapton PJ, O'Sullivan JP et al: Encephalopathy in acute leukaemia associated with methotrexate therapy. Arch Dis Child 47:344–354, 1972.

13. Hendin B, DeVivo DC, Torach R et al: Parenchymatous degeneration of the central nervous system in childhood leukemia. Cancer 33:468–482, 1974.

14. Borns PF, Rancier LF: Cerebral calcifications in childhood leukemia mimicking Sturge-Weber Syndrome. Am J Roentgenol 122:52–55, 1974.

15. Spehl MJ, Flament R et al: Diffuse intracranial calcification appearing during the follow-up of acute lymphoblastic leukemia. Ann Radiol (Paris)17:417–422, 1974.

16. Flament-Durand J, Ketelbant-Balasse P, Maurus R et al: Intracerebral calcifications appearing during the course of acute lymphocytic leukemia treated with methotrexate and X-rays. Cancer 35:319–325, 1975.

17. Michotte Y, Smeyers-Verbeke J et al: Brain calcification in a case of acute lymphoblastic leukaemia. J Neurol Sci 25:145–152, 1975.

18. Rubinstein LJ, Herman MM, Long TF, Wilbur JR: Disseminated necrotizing leukoencephalopathy; a complication of treated central nervous system leukemia and lymphoma. Cancer 35:291–305, 1975.

19. Moir DH, Bale PM: Necropsy findings in childhood leukemia, emphasizing neutropenic enterocolitis and cerebral calcification. Pathology 8:247–258, 1976.

20. Meadows AT, Evans AE: Effects of chemotherapy on the central nervous system; a study of parenteral methotrexate in long-term survivors of leukemia and lymphoma in childhood. Cancer 37:1079–1085, 1976.

21. Mueller S, Bell W, Seibert J: Cerebral calcifications associated with intrathecal methotrexate therapy in acute lymphocytic leukemia. J Pediatr 88:650–653, 1976.

22. DeVivo DC, Malas D, Nelson JS, Land VJ: Leukoencephalopathy in childhood leukemia. Neurology 27:609–613, 1977.

23. McIntosh S, Fischer DB, Rothman SG et al: Intracranial calcifications in childhood leukemia; an association with systemic chemotherapy. J Pediatr 91:909–913, 1977.

24. Price RA, Jamieson PA: The central nervous system in childhood leukemia. II. Subacute leukoencephalopathy. Cancer 35:306–318, 1975.

25. Price RA, Birdwell DA: The central nervous system in childhood leukemia. III. Mineralizing microangiopathy and dystrophic calcification. Cancer 42: 717–728, 1978.

26. Aur RJA, Simone JV, Verzosa MS et al: Childhood acute leukemia; Study VIII. Cancer 42:2123–2134, 1978.

27. Lee RC: Evolution in the concept of the blood-brain barrier phenomenon. In Progress in Neuropathology, Zimmerman HM (Ed). Grune & Stratton, New York, 1971, pp. 34–145.

28. Griffin TW, Rasey JS, Bleyer WA: The effect of photon irradiation on blood-brain barrier permeability to methotrexate in mice. Cancer 40:1109–1111, 1977.

29. Pincus JH, Reynolds GH, Glaser GH: Subacute combined system degeneration with folate deficiency. JAMA 221(5):496–497, 1972.

30. Price RA: Pathology of central-nervous-system diseases in childhood leukemia. In Neuro-Oncology, Clinical and Experimental Aspects, Ongerboer de Visser BW, Bosch DA, van Woerkom-Eykenboom WMH (Eds). Martinus Nijhoff Publishers, Boston, 1980, pp. 186–205.

10. Neurotoxic Complications of CNS prophylaxis in Childhood Leukaemia

M.G. MOTT

Introduction

There is general agreement that the biggest single advance in the treatment of childhood leukaemia in the last fifteen years has been the introduction of effective CNS prophylaxis against meningeal relapse, usually with a combination of cranial radiation and intrathecal methotrexate. With few exceptions this procedure has been adopted as standard in the last ten years and every Institution which sees a significant number of patients now has many long-term survivors who had cranial radiation and intrathecal prophylaxis as part of the treatment for their childhood acute lymphoblastic leukaemia (ALL). The long-term complications of the treatment process have become increasingly important as a consequence of the rising proportion of children with ALL who have been cured of their disease. Modifications of treatment regimens involve a delicate balance between seeking the maximum number of 'cures' while at the same time attempting to minimize the treatment sequelae which are the price that cured patients have to pay. The consequences of treatment are of particular importance when vital organs such as the brain are subjected to potentially harmful procedures as part of the treatment process. The observed long-term complications of irradiation for brain tumours include effects on intellectual performance and growth and development mediated by the hypothalamic-pituitary axis. These have led to a concern that such complications might also occur in leukaemic children who received the much smaller doses of radiation given for prophylaxis against meningeal leukaemia, but in combination with intrathecal drugs such as methotrexate. Our awareness of these potential complications led to a series of pilot studies on the CNS effects of treatment for childhood ALL in some of the first long-term survivors of the era of CNS prophylaxis, in order to determine whether we would have to re-evaluate the role of this mode of treatment. We studied first the intellectual performance of these children, then the integrity of their hypothalamic-pituitary axis, and lastly we looked for evidence of structural abnormalities in the brain which might be regarded as a consequence of treatment.

R. Mastrangelo, D.G. Poplack, R. Riccardi (eds), Central Nervous System Leukemia. ISBN 978-94-009-6710-6.
© *1983 Martinus Nijhoff Publishers, Boston.*

Intellectual function

A comprehensive psychological assessment (Wechsler Intelligence Scale for Children, WISC) was undertaken in 9 patients whose ages ranged from 8.8 to 15.9 years at the time of testing, some 4 to 7 years after their treatment with cranio-spinal radiation and intrathecal methotrexate. Evaluation of their full-scale, verbal and performance IQ together with reading age indicated that, with one exception, they were well within the normal range. The one exception was a child who performed poorly in the IQ test but who was known to have had a highly abnormal educational and social background during the preceding five years. This patient's subsequent progress has confirmed that she in fact performs at a level well above that recorded on the IQ test and strongly suggests that these readings are artifactual and do not truly represent her actual intellectual status.

It was apparent from this pilot study that there was no evidence of severe intellectual retardation in our patients and, given the very complex background of other factors which might also affect IQ performance in such patients, it was clear that much larger numbers of patients would be required to determine the factors related to impaired intellectual performance than we could provide in our Institution. These patients were in fact included in a multi-Institution study, the results of which have been published (1) and our later patients have also been included in more comprehensive studies, the results of which were presented at this symposium.

Hypothalamic-pituitary function

Fourteen children, of whom 8 were girls and 6 were boys, were studied when aged 6.9 to 15.2 years. They had all been in continuous complete remission for a minimum of 3.2. years (mean 5 years) and off all specific treatment for more than one year. They all had ALL diagnosed at a mean age of 5.4. years and all had been pre-pubertal at diagnosis. All had received cranio-spinal irradiation from an orthovoltage source receiving a mean of 2,100 rads to the cranium and an estimated 500–600 rads to the thyroid gland. Growth, puberty stage and skeletal age were assessed in all patients. Eight of the 14 children agreed to undergo a four hour combined hypothalamic-anterior pituitary function test (2) which involves the simultaneous intravenous injection of insulin (0.1 unit per kilogram), thyrotrophin releasing hormone (TRH 200 μg) and luteinising-hormone releasing hormone (LHRH 100 μg) after basal samples have been withdrawn through an indwelling 'butterfly' needle. Two hours after the insulin injection oral L-dopa is given as a second stimulus to growth hormone production. Results in these children were compared to the known range of normal values for children in our Centre.

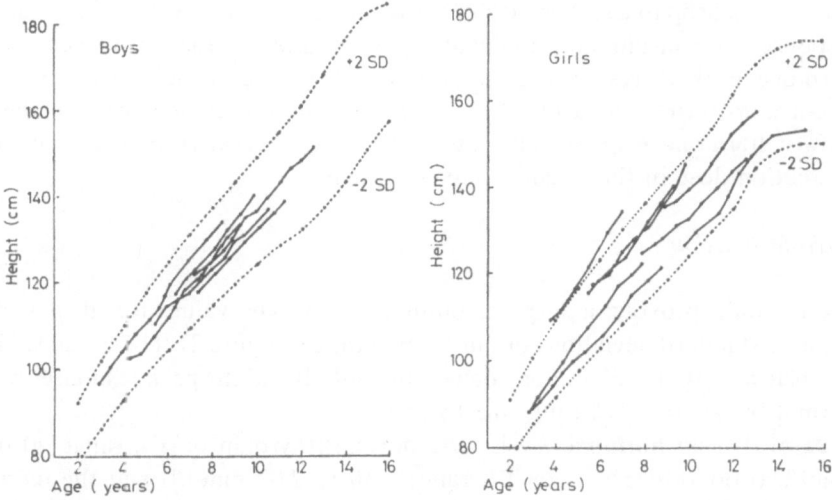

Figure 1. Growth curves of 14 children treated for ALL.

Anthropometric data

Growth charts for all 14 children show that none was of short stature and that linear growth was normal in all in relation to their age and stage of puberty (Figure 1). The stage of puberty and skeletal age were likewise normal in all patients.

Growth velocity curves showed that growth velocity may be sub-optimal during maintenance treatment but that there is a catch-up growth spurt in these children in the year after treatment is completed. In the 12 children who were still pre-pubertal, mean growth velocity was 5.9 cms per year (range 4.6 to 8.6) in the year preceding cessation of therapy and 7.2 cms per year (range 5.0 to 9.2) in the year after treatment was discontinued. This certainly suggests that treatment may suppress growth to some extent but the recovery after chemotherapy is discontinued seems inconsistent with long-term damage to the production of growth hormone.

Endocrine evaluation

Growth hormone

Using the test described above normally growing children achieve a peak hormone response of at least 8.0 mU/l during the test procedure. The peak levels achieved by the leukaemic children all exceeded this minimal response. Hypoglycaemia, defined as a drop to less than 50% of the resting blood sugar value, was achieved in response to the insulin injection in all 8 patients and 6 of the 8 produced a growth hormone peak in response of >8 mU/l. All 8 children achieved >8 mU/l in response to their L-dopa (Table 1). We found no correlation between the peak growth hormone response and either the time interval from radiation or the irradiation dose in this small group of patients.

Thyroid function

TRH should provoke a surge of pituitary TSH. The values for all patients lie within 2 standard deviations of our normal range (Figure 2). The basal TSH level was below 3 mU/l in all but one patient (4.5 mU/l) and the peak responses were all normal (mean 14 mU/l range 6.2 to 15 mU/l).

Basal thyroid hormone levels were normal (thyroxin or T4, range 70 to 115 nmol/l, trioodothyronene or T3, range 1.10 to 2.02 nmol/l) and the increment achieved after two hours of TRH injection confirmed competent thyroid gland activity (mean T4 increment 16%, mean T3 increment 38%).

Cortisol

All the children had basal or stimulated levels of plasma cortisol above 400 nmol/l, indicating adequate hypothalamic-pituitary adrenal responses to stress. The basal range was 250 to 905 nmol/l (8.9 to 32.3 μg/100 ml). Responses to hypoglycaemia were satisfactory in those with normal basal levels but no response was seen when the basal level was above 600 nmol/l (21.4 μg/100 ml). The range of cortisol levels sixty minutes after insulin was 425 to 725 nmol/l (15.1 to 25.8 μg/100 ml).

Table 1. Peak GH response following insulin and L-DOPA.

Case Number	GH peak response mU/l		Max GH peak mU/l
	Insulin	L-DOPA	
1	7.3	9.4	9.4
2	8.7	16.7	16.7
3	21.0	14.1	21.0
4	11.6	13.4	13.4
5	11.1	13.1	13.1
6	6.1	14.4	14.4
7	14.3	8.3	14.3
8	27.6	36.6	36.6
Mean	13.5	16.2	17.4

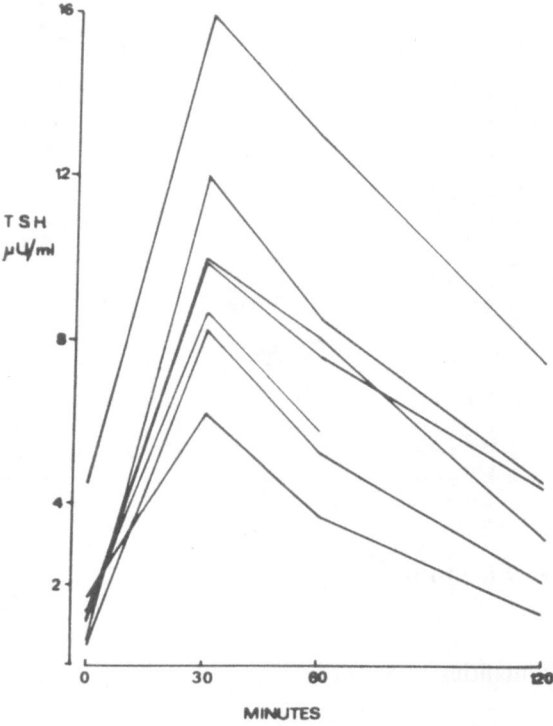

Figure 2. TSH response to TRH.

Gonadotrophins and gonadal steroids

Release of luteinising hormone (LH) is provoked by injected LHRH and the response in all our patients was consistent with the child's pubertal status and age (Figure 3). LH levels rose from low basal levels (maximum 3.3. units/l) to a mean peak at thirty minutes of 17.2 units/l (range 7.6 to 24.3 units/l). The maximum response in the pre-pubertal children was 6.9 units/l. One fully pubertal, normally menstruating girl had a rather blunted response with a peak LH of 7.6 units/l which was fully consistent with the follicular phase of her menstrual cycle at the time of testing (3).

The FSH responses were all within the range seen in normal children. There was no rise in serum testosterone or oestradiol in the pre-pubertal children four hours following LHRH but satisfactory increments of gonadal steroids were seen in all 5 of the pubertal children. The 2 pubertal boys showed a satisfactory rise is serum testosterone and the 3 pubertal girls a similar increment in their oestradiol levels.

88

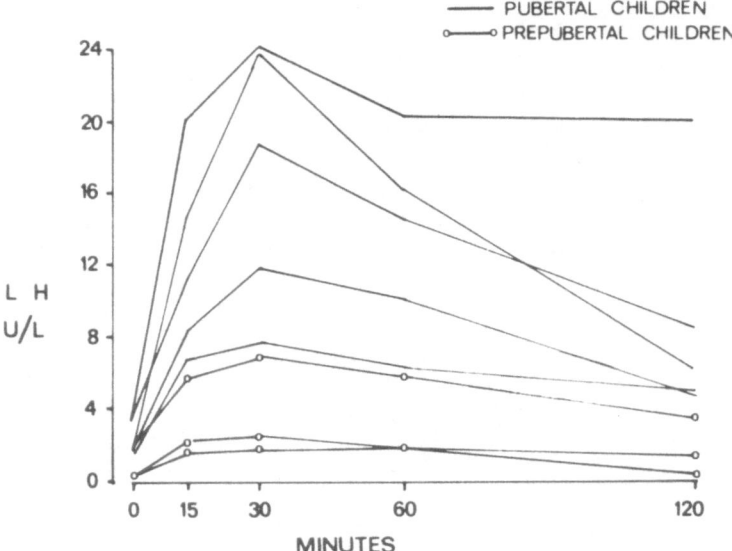

PUBERTAL CHILDREN
PREPUBERTAL CHILDREN

Figure 3. LH response to LHRH.

Structural abnormalities

Forty-two patients, whose treatment for ALL or T cell leukaemia/lymphoma included cranal radiation and intrathecal methotrexate were investigated by means of computerized axial tomography (CAT) of the brain (Table 2). Most patients had received orthovoltage radiation to a mean dose of 2,100 rads to the cranium in 10 to 15 fractions over eleven to twenty-two days, a dose which is supposedly biologically equivalent to 2,500 rads from a megavoltage source with the same fractionation. Intrathecal methotrexate was given in various schedules to these patients to a mean total dose of 62.5 mgms/m², the largest dose given over the longest period being to 6 children on the UKALL I schedule who received 10 mgs/m² × 11 doses between weeks 17 and 55 of treatment. A group of 7 patients received intermittent orthovoltage radiation given in eight monthly fractions, to a total of 2,000 rads with intrathecal methotrexate given each time on the same day. A further 7 patients with T cell disease received a dose of 1,760 rads in eight fractions over a ten day period from a megavoltage source (1.25 meV) or its biological equivalent from the orthovoltage machine.

None of the children investigated had developed meningeal disease during the course of their treatment and at the time of CAT scan all were in remission and attending normal school with one exception, a patient known to be developmentally retarded before his leukaemia was diagnosed.

Quantitative assessment of ventricular size was attempted in the largest group of 28 patients by the method of Hahn and Rim (4). The diameter of the frontal

Table 2.

Treatment Protocol	Age at Treatment (yrs)	Interval RT-CT (mo)	Radiation			
			Source	Dose (rads)	Fractions	Time (days)
Standard A.L.L.	1.3–11 (5.8)	20–84 (52)	250 Kv	2100	10–15	11–22
Intermittent A.L.L.	3.9–11.5 (6.4)	16–23 (20)	250 Kv	2000	× 8	8 months
T cell	6–14 (10.3)	3–32 (18)	250 Kv	1800	8	9–13
			1.25 meV	1760	8	9–10

horns was measured and compared with the diameter of the brain at the same point giving (i) the bi-frontal ratio through the anterior corner and (ii) the bicaudate ratio through the body of the frontal horns at the level of the caudate nucleus. A second assessment of ventricular size was made using the method described by Enzmann and Lane (5).

Results

None of the scans showed areas of calcification and only one contained abnormal areas of low density as described by Ramu *et al.* 1978 (6). Subjectively, it appeared that the sulci or subarachnoid spaces were more obvious in some patients than in others but in none of these were the findings considered to be definitely outside of the normal range. The one child who was known to be abnormal before diagnosis, having been born prematurely and with documented low intelligence before treatment, was found to have moderately dilated ventricles on his scan. His intellectual performance has not deteriorated since the diagnosis of acute lymphoblastic leukaemia and it does not seem reasonable therefore to attribute his ventricular dilatation to his treatment. Results of the measurements of the ventricles of the other 27 patients in Group 1 are all within the normal range, with the exception of 1 patient whose bifrontal diameter is separated from the rest though still within the upper limit of normal (Figure 4). The ventricles of this patient are considered enlarged by the criteria of Enzmann and Lane. This patient received 2,000 rads radiation and only 22 mgm/m^2 of intrathecal methotrexate. She had extensive retinal haemorrhages at diagnosis and the rounding of the frontal horns on her scan may possibly be regarded as abnormal.

The children receiving intermittent monthly doses of cranial radiation together with intrathecal methotrexate and those having the smaller dose of 1,760 rads for T cell disease likewise show no structural abnormalities on CAT scanning with

90

one exception (Figure 5). The patient was one of three T cell patients who received megavoltage rather than orthovoltage radiation because he had been randomized to receive radiation to his mediastinum concurrently with his cranial radiation. His CAT scan 6 months post cranial radiation shows some of the abnormalities described by Ramu *et al.*, with a marked improvement 6 months later.

Discussion

Although the number of patients we have investigated is small, we have found no convincing evidence that the cranial radiation and intrathecal therapy as given in our Centre has caused long-term damage to the CNS. The results are similar to those reported from several other Centres but are at variance with other reports, where pathological changes in intellectual function, hypothalamic-pituitary axis function and structural brain abnormalities have all been documented. The reason for this apparent discrepancy between Centres is not clear. It is important to stress

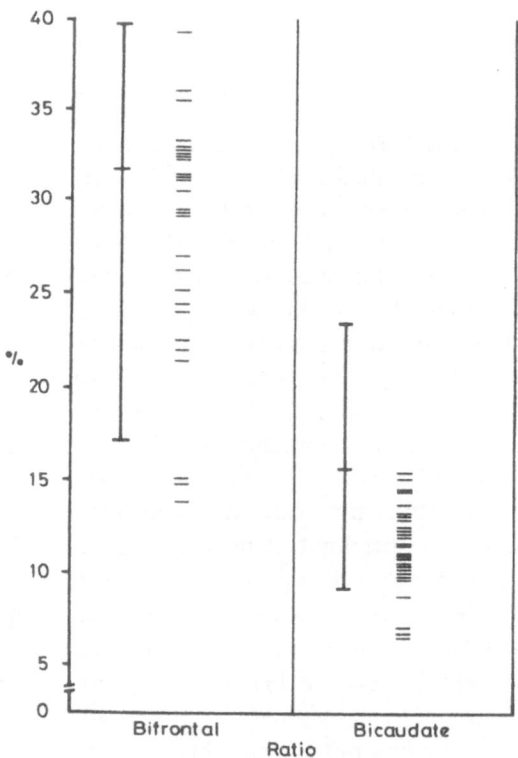

Figure 4. Ventricle/brain ratios in 27 children compared to mean and range in normal adults.

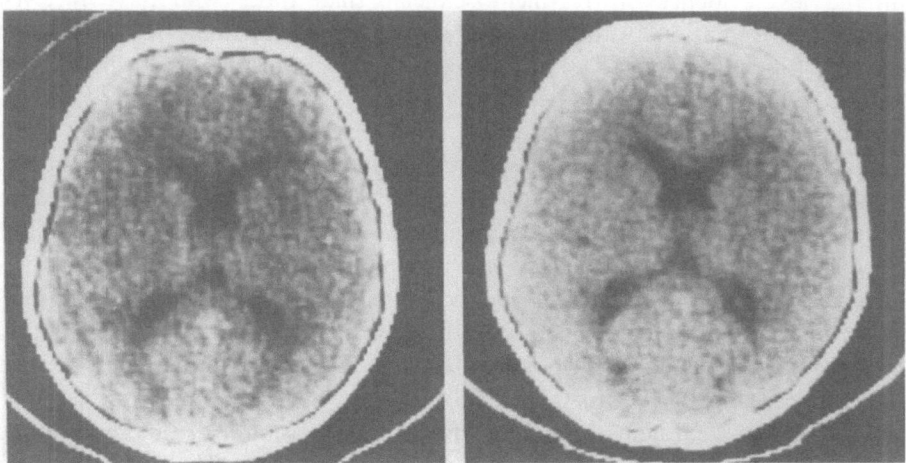

Figure 5. CT scans 6 and 12 months after megavoltage radiation.

that the CNS prophylaxis offered to children with leukaemia in terms of cranial radiation and intrathecal therapy varies considerably from one centre to another. The most obvious difference between the treatment given to the patients described in this report and that given in those reports documenting many abnormalities is our use of orthovoltage as opposed to megavoltage radiation. The reason for our choice of orthovoltage radiation has been purely pragmatic. The linear accelerators betatron and cobalt units in our Radiation Therapy Centre are used much more intensively than the orthovoltage machine. Accurate radiotherapy to the cranium in children requires a careful setup and considerable cooperation from the patient to lie still, and this is not easily achieved with the young patients. Many Centres resort to sedation or even anaesthesia in order to give accurate radiation to their children, but we do our best to avoid this. The period of cranial radiation usually comes about one month after the illness is first diagnosed, when, for the first time, they are beginning to feel well and are over the immediate complications that arise during induction therapy. I believe that it is psychologically most important to have the child as well as possible during this time, from their own point of view and that of their parents, to reinforce the notion that they may expect to lead a relatively normal life once the disease is under control. A consequence of the determination to avoid sedation or anaesthesia, however, is that the radiotherapy technicians have to spend a considerable amount of time playing with the children and acclimatizing them to the apparatus before they are able to get sufficient cooperation to give them their radiation therapy safely and correctly. This is the reason that we have opted for the use of the orthovoltage machine which in turn may be the reason why these patients appear to have suffered less evidence of treatment sequelae than those who have received megavoltage radiation. Another factor that is almost certainly relevant is the amount of intrathecal medication given and the length of time over which this is prescribed. In a number of studies in which longterm damage has been described, maintenance intrathecal chemotherapy was given over many months. The treatment of childhood leukemia is complex and involves many changes in the child's environment in addition to the potentially toxic therapy prescribed to control the disease. The emotional and educational problems alone might well be considered to be of sufficient severity to lead to suboptimal intellectual performance once treatment has been completed. It is in fact remarkable how normal most children are after they have been through such a traumatic process. Of all the many factors which might possibly result in intellectual impairment, the one which appears most critical is the age of the child when radiation takes place (1), and the current treatment regimen in the UK takes account of this by delaying prophylactic cranial radiation until after the second birthday. The most important factor in the endocrine studies appears to be the precise dose and fractionation of the radiation administered (9). The widely different frequency of abnormalities detected by CT scanning of the brain in different series seems likely also to be related to the type and dose/fractionation of radiation and the frequency and duration of intrathecal therapy. Some of the findings are largely subjective and are difficult to quantify. The amount of fluid appearing in the sulci and subarachnoid space, for example, varies widely in the normal population and can alter substantially in the same patient depending on such simple factors as the state of hydration. Differences in climate and management policy e.g. whether children are kept nil by mouth and/or are anaesthetised for CT scanning might therefore account for some of the observed differences, and caution should be exercised in extrapolating from observed deviations from the norm to implying the presence of organic brain damage.

A recent report suggests that the dose of cranial radiation may safely be reduced from 2,400 rads to 1,800 rads for a substantial majority of children with acute lymphoblastic leukaemia without loss of efficacy in terms of the degree of control of meningeal disease (6). It is also possible that we may now be able to identify specific groups of patients whose risk of meningeal relapse is low enough that it is reasonable to consider attempting treatment for them without the use of cranial radiation. The only mature study to date in which children treated without the use of cranial radiation have had a comparable low incidence of CNS relapse is the report from Memorial Hospital of the L2 protocol, which is an intensive multidrug chemotherapy that includes many agents which cross the blood brain barrier and have presumably been effective in eradicating meningeal foci in the place of radiation therapy (7). Results of other studies, using for example intermediate doses of intravenous methotrexate instead of cranial radiation as CNS prophylaxis have shown an increased incidence of CNS leukaemia, as the studies have matured, so that early hopes that this might be a suitable alternative have been disappointed (8).

On present evidence it would appear that prophylactic cranial radiation and intrathecal methotrexate remain an essential part of the therapy of most children with childhood acute lymphoblastic leukaemia. Studies of long-term survivors treated in the seventies suggest that the therapy used may have been sufficient to cause long-term abnormalities in some of the survivors. The reduction in the dose of radiation now shown to give adequate CNS prophylaxis suggests that this problem should be minimal for those patients who will be receiving these lower doses in the future.

References

1. Eiser C: Intellectual abilities among survivors of childhood leukaemia as a function of CNS irradiation. Arch Dis Childh 53:391–395, 1978.
2. Savage DCL, Swift RGF, Johnston PGB, Goldie DJ, Murphy D: Combined test of anterior pituitary function in children. Arch Dis Childh 53:301–304, 1978.
3. McNeilly AS, Hagen C: Prolactin. TSH, LH and FSH responses to a combined LHRH/TRH test at different stages of the menstrual cycle. Clin Endocrinol 3:427–435, 1974.
4. Hahn FSY, Rim K: Frontal ventricular dimensions on normal computer tomography. Am J Roentgenol, Radium Ther. and Nuclear Med 126:593, 1976.
5. Enzmann DR, Lane B: Cranial computed tomographic findings in anorexia nervosa. J Computer Assisted Tomography 1:140, 1977.
6. Nesbit M et al: Presymptomatic CNS Therapy in previously untreated Childhood ALL comparison of 1800 rad and 2400 rad. Lancet 1:461–465, 1981.
7. Haghbin M et al: A long term clinical follow up of children with ALL treated with intensive chemotherapy regimens. Cancer 46:241–252, 1980.
8. Green D et al: Comparison of 3 methods of CNS prophylaxis in childhood ALL. Lancet 1:1398–1401, 1980.
9. Shalet S et al: Growth hormone deficiency after treatment of acute leukaemia in children. Arch Dis Childh 51:489–493, 1976.

11. Evaluation of Adverse Sequelae of Central Nervous System Prophylaxis in Acute Lymphoblastic Leukemia

D.G. POPLACK

Introduction

In recent years attention has focused on the potential for the development of adverse sequelae of central nervous system preventive therapy in children with acute lymphoblastic leukemia. Anatomic abnormalities (defined by CT brain scan), neuroendocrine damage, as well as neurological and intellectual dysfunction have all been reported in patients who have received central nervous system propvlaxis, usually in the form of cranial radiation and intrathecal chemotherapy. In the late 1970's the Pediatric Oncology Branch of the National Cancer Institute embarked on a series of studies designed to characterize the adverse sequelae associated with CNS prophylaxis (1–3). The present report will summarize the findings of these studies and discuss their implications for the treatment of the patient with ALL.

Our initial studies were performed on a group of asymptomatic acute lymphoblastic leukemia patients, all of whom were in continuous complete remission and had been treated on the same therapeutic protocol. Induction therapy consisted of systemic POMP (prednisone, vincristine, methotrexate and 6-mercaptopurine). Once complete remission was achieved, all patients received central nervous system preventive therapy which consisted of cranial radiation for all patients, and either intrathecal methotrexate or intrathecal cytosine arabinoside. The type of intrathecal chemotherapy was determined by randomization. The cranial radiation was delivered from a 6 MEV linear accelerator in 200 rad per day fractions to a total dose of 2400 rad. Intrathecal chemotherapy during the period of cranial radiation consisted of either 5 doses of methotrexate ($12 \ mg/m^2$) or 8 doses of cytosine arabinoside (Ara-C) ($30 \ mg/m^2$). Monthly intrathecal maintenance chemotherapy was given for a total period of 30 months. Maintenance systemic chemotherapy consisted of 6-mercaptopurine, methotrexate, vincristine and prednisone, all of which was continued for a total duration of 36 months.

In an attempt to define the adverse sequelae of this form of central nervous system preventive therapy, a comprehensive evaluation of those patients treated on this protocol who remained in continuous complete remission was instituted in

R. Mastrangelo, D.G. Poplack, R. Riccardi (eds), Central Nervous System Leukemia. ISBN 978-94-009-6710-6.
© *1983 Martinus Nijhoff Publishers, Boston.*

96

late 1976. Evaluation procedures included CT brain scans, detailed neurological examination, psychometric testing and neuroendocrine evaluation.

CT brain scans

In a previous study of a group of patients with clinically overt necrotizing leukoencephalopathy, we had determined that that syndrome was characterized by distinctive CT scan abnormalities which included areas of decreased attenuation coefficient (hypodensity of white matter), and the presence of intracerebral calcifications (4). The results of that study raised the question of whether similar CT scan abnormalities might be found in asymptomatic patients who had been treated with central nervous system preventive therapy. Thirty-two patients who had been treated on the protocol described above were in complete remission and available for CT scan study. Fourteen of these patients had received intrathecal methotrexate; 18 had received intrathecal Ara-C. Both groups were comparable with regards to age and sex, and there was no significant difference in the interval from the initiation of central nervous system preventive therapy to the time of CT scanning (23–67 months, median of 42 months, in the methotrexate group, and 19–63 months, median of 38 months, in the cytosine arabinoside group). The CT scans were performed with two EMI headscanners. Four patients were studied with the Mark I; all remaining patients were studied with a high resolution CT1010 model. Surprisingly, more than half (53%) of these asymptomatic patients demonstrated one or more of four CT scan abnormalities which included ventricular dilatation, dilatation of the subarachnoid space, areas of decreased attenuation coefficient (hypodense, abnormally radiolucent regions) and intracerebral calcifications (Figure 1). Of note was the fact that ventricular

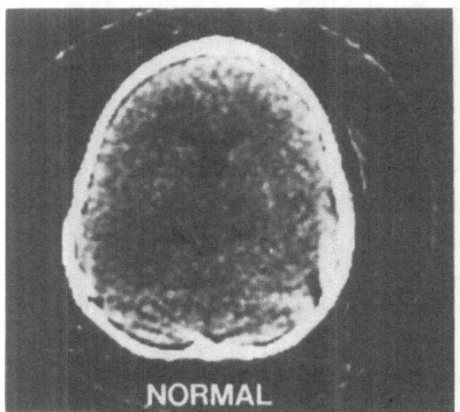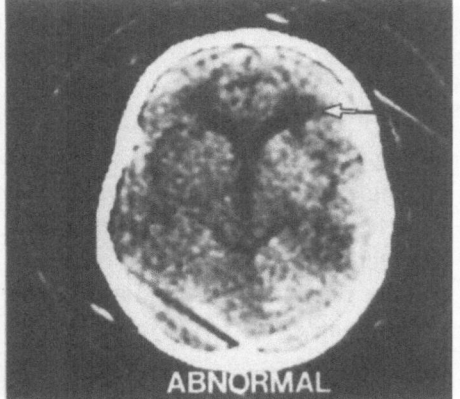

A

Figure 1A. CT scan demonstrating areas of deceased attenuation coefficient in periventricular regions (see arrow).

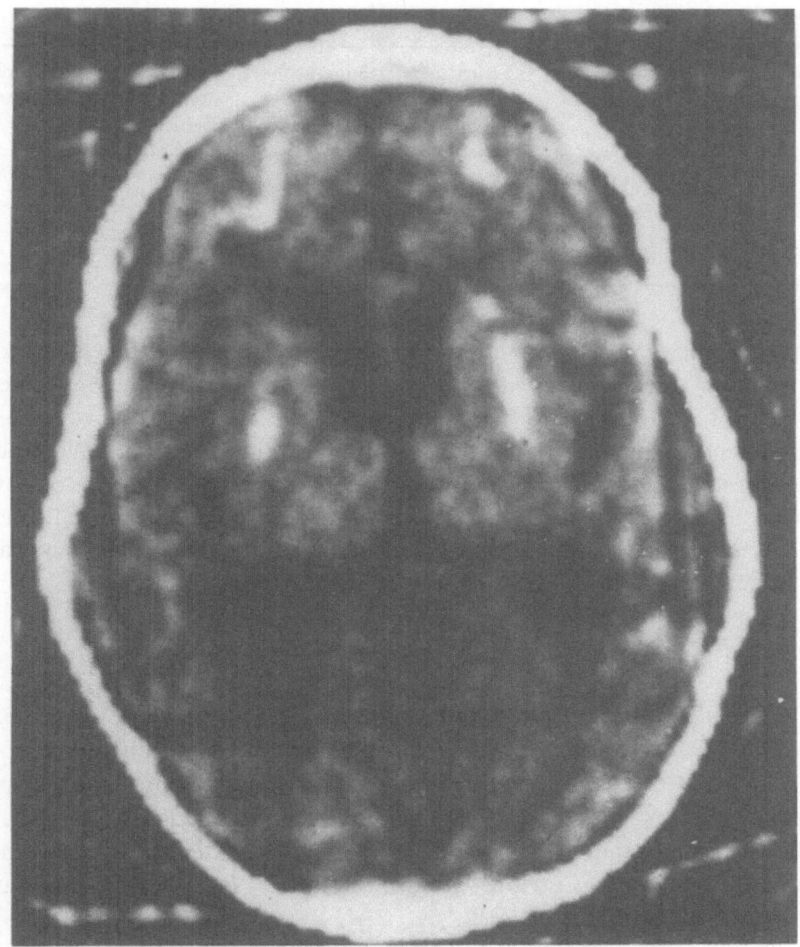

B

Figure 1B. CT scan demonstrating intracerebral calcifications.

dilatation and widening of the subarachnoid spaces were distributed among patients in both intrathecal chemotherapy groups, suggesting a relationship with central nervous system radiation (the CNS treatment received by all patients in this study). These types of lesions are believed to reflect cerebral cortical atrophy. Similar lesions have been pathologically confirmed in monkeys that have been treated with cranial radiation (5). In contrast, two other lesions, decreased attenuation coefficient in the periventricular regions (hypodensity of the white matter presumed to indicate demyelinization) and intracerebral calcification were found only in patients who received intrathecal methotrexate chemotherapy (Table 1). As noted previously, these lesions were also observed in 'methotrexate' leukoencephalopathy (necrotizing leukoencephalopathy).

Table 1. CT-scan abnormalities following CNS prophylaxis.

IT medication	No. of abn./ Total pts.	Ventricular dilatation	Subarachnoid space dilatation	Decreased attenuation coefficient	Intracerebral calcification
MTX	8/14	4	3	4	1
ARA-C	9/18	4	6	0	0
Total	17/32	8	9	4	1

As part of the same study, a control group of 11 patients with acute leukemia who had never received any central nervous system preventive therapy were also studied by CT scanning. The CT scan findings in this control group were normal.

The presence of unanticipated CT scan findings in a group of asymptomatic patients who had received central nervous system preventive therapy is of obvious concern, raising the possibility that these lesions represent 'preclinical' findings which eventually may be associated with clinically demonstrable sequelae. A longitudinal, long-term follow-up study of these patients is in progress.

Neurological evaluation

All of the patients in this study underwent comprehensive neurological examination (1). More than half of the patients manifested peripheral neurologic findings (e.g., decreased tendon reflexes) which were the presumed result of vincristine treatment. Seven patients manifested truncal ataxia, two of these also had lateral gaze nystagmus. None of these findings correlated with the presence or absence of CT scan abnormalities or with the type of intrathecal chemotherapy which these patients had received.

Psychometric testing

The effects of central nervous system prophylaxis on the intellectual function of this patient group was also evaluated. The Wechsler intelligence tests and the Bender-Gestalt tests of perceptual motor function were administered to these children and to control groups which consisted of both an age matched sample of their healthy sibling, and a group of patients with ALL who had never received any form of central nervous system therapy and their healthy siblings. The results of these studies revealed that the patients with leukemia who received central nervous system prophylaxis manifested significantly lower scores than their healthy sibling controls (2). The differences in IQ between these patients and their siblings was statistically significant ($p < 0.001$) for the comparison involving the full scale, verbal scale and performance scale IQ's. The mean IQ scores for the patients averaged approximately 99 versus 113 for the healthy siblings (Table 2).

Table 2. Comparison of Wechsler intelligence test results in leukemia patients and healthy siblings.

	Mean full scale IQ	Mean verbal scale IQ	Mean performance scale IQ
CNS treated patients	98.6	99.9	97.8
Siblings	112.5	112.2	110.0
IQ difference	− 13.9*	− 12.3*	− 12.2*

* P value less than 0.001 level of significance based on two tailed t tests for correlated means.

According to the Wechsler test manual, these scores would place the patients at the 47th, and the siblings at the 79th percentile ranks. This difference between the patient and the sibling groups is believed sufficient to have bearing on the patient's potential for academic achievement. Furthermore, the results of the Wechsler sub-test scores revealed that the CNS treated patients differed significantly from their siblings in tests which measured associative thinking, remote memory, the ability to utilize and manipulate abstract concepts, awareness of details, and the capacity for perceptual analysis, organization and synthesis. The findings from the Bender-Gestalt test of perceptual motor functioning were consistent with the IQ results. In contrast to the differences between the CNS treated patients and their siblings, no differences were seen on these tests between the ALL patients who never received CNS prophylaxis and their siblings, or between a third control group of cystic fibrosis patients and a group of their healthy siblings. This study also revealed that those patients who received central nervous system preventive treatment at a younger age exhibited a greater decrement in intellectual abilities than did patients who were older at the time of treatment.

Hypothalamic-pituitary function studies

The patient group was also studied to assess the status of their hypothalamic-pituitary function following CNS prophylaxis. The possibility of neuroendocrine damage in these individuals had been suggested by previous studies in which abnormal growth hormone responses to provocative stimuli such as insulin-induced hypoglycemia had been observed in patients receiving cranial radiation and intrathecal chemotherapy (6, 7).

All patients received a comprehensive neuroendocrine work-up. Intravenous insulin, LHRH and TRH were given as provocative stimuli for the release of growth hormone, cortisol, FSH, LH, TSH, T_3 and prolactin. In addition, posterior pituitary function was also studied. The only significant abnormality noted was a decreased growth hormone response to insulin-induced hypoglycemia which occurred in 50% of the patients who received CNS prophylaxis. In contrast, all other parameters of anterior pituitary and hypothalamic function were normal.

Interestingly, there was a significant correlation between abnormally low peak growth hormone responses and ventricular dilatation on CT scans. Of the 23 patients available for testing, 7 of the 9 patients with abnormally low growth hormone responses also demonstrated ventricular dilatation on CT brain scans, whereas only 1 of the 9 patients with normal growth hormone responses demonstrated the CT scan finding (Figure 2). Since, as mentioned above, ventricular dilatation is believed to be an adverse effect of cranial radiation, the correlation noted in this study is consistent with the hypothesis that abnormal growth hormone responses may be due to an adverse effect of radiotherapy upon

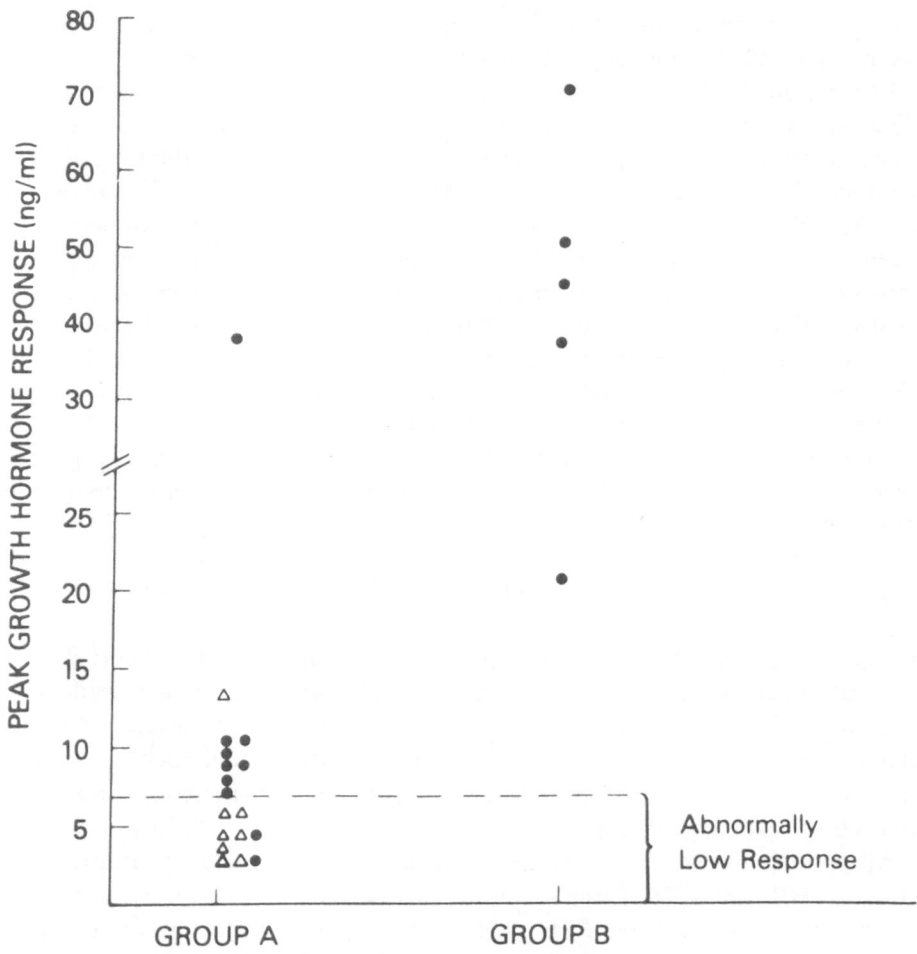

Figure 2. Peak growth hormone responses during insulin tolerance testing and the presence of ventricular dilatation. Group A, patients treated with cranial radiation and intrathecal chemotherapy on Protocol 72–1; Group B, a small group of patients with acute lymphocytic leukemia who have received systemic chemotherapy but no CNS prophylaxis.

the hypothalamic-pituitary axis. Although it was not possible to definitively rule out a contributory role for either systemic or intrathecal chemotherapy in the development of the abnormal growth hormone response, it is of interest that no such abnormalities were noted in a small group of patients with ALL who had never received central nervous system prophylaxis. The clinical implications of the abnormal growth hormone responses are not completely clear. There was no clear correlation between the abnormally low growth hormone responses and short stature.

Discussion

The comprehensive evaluation of this group of asymptomatic ALL patients who had undergone central nervous system prophylaxis revealed the presence of abnormalities on CT brain scans, and in neurologic, psychometric and hypothalamic-pituitary function testing.

The finding of CT scan abnormalities in more than half of the patients evaluated provides definitive evidence of therapy-related CNS structural damage. Although there was no correlation between the presence of these CT scan abnormalities and the neurological dysfunction noted, it remains unclear whether the presence of these lesions portends the possibility of overt clinical symptomatology at some point in the future. These patients are being carefully followed in an effort to determine whether overt clinical symtomatology becomes manifest. It is important to note that patients in this study received monthly intrathecal maintenance therapy for a total of 30 months, a more intensive regimen of central nervous system preventive therapy than many currently in use. It is possible that regimens utilizing less intensive intrathecal chemotherapy and/or lower doses of cranial radiation may not be accompanied by as high an incidence of CT scan changes. The subsequent clinical experience of other investigators (some of which is presented elsewhere in this book) appears to support this thesis. In this regard, it is of interest that in a subsequent study of another patient group given CNS prophylaxis with a lower dose of cranial radiation (2000 rad), and only a singly dose of intrathecal chemotherapy, no abnormal CT scan findings were noted (8).

The results of the psychometric studies are of obvious concern. Our data strongly suggest that central nervous system preventive therapy may have a significant adverse effect on the intellectual capability of children with acute lymphoblastic leukemia. The results of our study established that a decrement in intellectual functioning occurred between the time of initiation of central nervous system treatment and the time of initial psychological testing. It is of interest that the IQ scores obtained upon follow-up testing one year later were not significantly different from those scores obtained initially, suggesting that the deterioration in intellectual functioning may not be progressive beyond a certain point. To what extent the deterioration in intellectual functioning reflects the intensity of the prophylaxis regimen utilized in these patients is unclear. However, it is notable that other investigators have also demonstrated abnormalities in the intellectual abilities of survivors of acute lymphoblastic leukemia who received more conventional, less intensive CNS preventive therapy (9, 10). Clearly the results of our studies emphasize the need for comprehensive psychometric evaluation of all patients receiving central nervous system preventive therapy. It is possible that early identification of patients with similar deficits and rapid intervention with specialized, compensatory education may have remedial benefits. Our results also suggest the importance of a prospective, longitudinal psychometric evaluation of patients undergoing CNS prophylaxis. Such a study is under way in our institution.

The studies of hypothalamic-pituitary function in this patient group indicated that central nervous system preventive therapy can adversely effect the hypothalamic-pituitary axis and that CT brain scanning may be of value in predicting which patients will exhibit this abnormality. However, there was no clear cut correlation between the presence of an abnormal growth hormone response to insulin-induced hypoglycemia and patient growth. Nevertheless, the finding of hypothalamic-pituitary damage also emphasizes the need to search for equally effective, but less toxic methods of CNS preventive therapy. It is notable that, in a subsequent study, we have documented that a smaller total dose of cranial radiation is not accompanied by neuroendocrine abnormalities (8).

In summary, the above studies have documented the potential of CNS preventive therapy to produce adverse CNS sequelae. Recognition of this potential is crucial for the clinician who follows patients treated with similar preventive CNS therapy. The obvious immediate challenge to the pediatric oncology community is to formulate equally effective CNS prophylactic regimens which are not associated with these types of CNS damage.

References

1. Peylan-Ramu N, Poplack DG, Pizzo PA, Adornato BT, Di Chiro G: Abnormal CT scans of the brain in asymptomatic children with acute lymphocytic leukemia after prophylactic treatment of the central nervous system with radiation and intrathecal chemotherapy. N Engl J Med 298:845-818, 1978.
2. Moss HA, Nannis ED, Poplack DG: The effects of prophylactic treatment of the central nervous system on the intellectual functioning of children with acute lymphocytic leukemia. Am J Med 71:47-52, 1981.
3. Oliff A, Bode U, Bercu B, DiChiro G, Graves V, Poplack DG: Hypothalamic-pituitary dysfunction following CNS prophylaxis in acute lymphocytic leukemia. Med and Pediatr Oncol 7:141-151, 1979.
4. Peylan-Ramu N, Poplack DG, Blei LC, Herdt JR, Vermess M, DiChiro G: Computer assisted tomography in methotrexate encephalopathy. J Compt Assist Tomogr, Vol. 1, pp. 216-221, April, 1977.

5. Caveness WF: Pathology of radiation damage to the normal brain of the monkey: Symposium on modern concepts in brain tumor therapy. Natl Cancer Inst Monogr 46:57–76, 1977.
6. Shalet SM, Beardwell CG, Twomey PH, Jones PHM, Pearson D: Endocrine function following the treatment of acute leukemia in childhood. J Pediatr 90:920–923, 1977.
7. Dickinson WP, Berry DH, Dickinson L *et al*: Differential effects of cranial radiation on growth hormone response to arginine and insulin. J Pediatr 92:745–747, 1978.
8. Bode U, Oliff A, Bercu B, DiChiro G, Glaubiger D, Poplack DG: Absence of CT brain scan and endocrine abnormalities with less intensive CNS prophylaxis. Am J Ped Hemat Oncol 2:21–24, 1980.
9. Obetz SW, Smithson WS, Gruber RV, *et al*: Neuropsychological follow-up study of central nervous system function in children with acute lymphocytic leukemia. Proc Am Soc Clin Oncol 20:342, 1979.
10. Meadows AT, Gordon J, Littman P *et al*: Pattern of cognitive dysfunctions in children with acute lymphocytic leukemia treated with cranial radiation. Proc Am Soc Clin Oncol 21:385, 1980.

12. Adverse Sequelae of Central Nervous System Prophylaxis in Acute Lymphoblastic Leukemia

G. PAOLUCCI and P. ROSITO

Introduction

Using currently available optimal therapy, approximately 50% of patients with Acute Lymphoblastic Leukemia (ALL) will be disease-free 5 years after diagnosis. Critical to successful therapy is the prevention of clinically undetectable leukemic involvement of the Central Nervous System (CNS). Although multiple methods of CNS Preventive Therapy (CNS prophylaxis) have been attempted, craniospinal or cranial irradiation plus methotrexate (MTX) have been proved effective and are most widely used.

With increasing numbers of ALL patients surviving, attention has focused on long-term therapy related sequelae, particularly of the CNS. Both acute neurologic toxicity (11) and chronic neurologic dysfunction have been reported by many investigators. The most severe form is leukoencephalopathy (1, 3, 11, 20, 22), a clinicopathologic entity which is characterized by irritability, confusion, ataxia and slurred speech which ultimately may progress to dementia, seizures and death. Brain necroscopy findings (4, 14, 20) consist of discrete multifocal areas of necrosis randomly disseminated in the cerebral white matter, axonal degeneration and astrocytosis, and scattered mineralized gray matter lesions. The incidence of this delayed neurologic syndrome is variable and appears to depend on the type of therapy (1); treatment regimens which include CNS irradiation appear to be the most neurotoxic.

Another form of delayed neuropathology described by Price (19) is mineralizing microangiopathy with dystrophic calcifications. Unlike leukoencephalopathy this desease predominantly affects the gray matter of the CNS. Price has proposed that the susceptibility of the microvasculature to adverse effects of ionizing radiation is the principal factor in the development of this lesion. Of additional concern is that abnormalities of Computed Tomography (CT) brain scans have been found in asymptomatic disease-free children with ALL. Subtle CNS dysfunction also has been revealed by means of EEG and neuropsychological studies in these children.

Concern regarding the late toxicity of CNS prophylaxis prompted us to study a group of 36 children with ALL off-therapy by means of CT brain scans, EEG and psychometric tests.

R. Mastrangelo, D.G. Poplack, R. Riccardi (eds), Central Nervous System Leukemia. ISBN 978-94-009-6710-6.
© 1983 Martinus Nijhoff Publishers, Boston.

Patients and methods

Thirty-six patients (18 boys and 18 girls) with the diagnosis of ALL, admitted to the Department of Pediatrics of the University of Bologna between 1972 and 1978, were included in this study. Patient ages ranged from 1.3 to 9.6 (median 4.2) years at diagnosis. Twenty-one children were aged <5 years (6 were 1–2 years old) and 15 were aged ≥ 5 years. No patient had CNS leukemia at diagnosis. The follow-up time for these patients is 3.7–8.9 years (median 5.4). At the time of the present study patient ages ranged from 6 to 16 years (median 9 years). All patients were in their first remission and all were off-therapy from 0.5 to 4 years (median 2.1 years). The interval from the end of cranial irradiation to the time of the study ranged from 3.5 to 7 years (median 4.2 years).

Induction therapy for most of the patients consisted of prednisone and vincristine. Maintenance systemic chemotherapy with daily 6-mercaptopurine and weekly IM MTX (20 mg/m^2) and pulses of prednisone and vincristine (every 3 months) were administered for a total of 36 months in 31 children and 48 months in the remaining 5.

Cranial irradiation was delivered through two opposite portals using a ^{60}Co unit; the dose at the midline of the brain was 130–147 rad per day; the total dose was 1890–2072 rad in 6 children (≤2 years old) and 2390–2550 in the remaining patients. In all children cranial irradiation was delivered early in remission, within 2 months from initial diagnosis. All the patients received intrathecal (IT) chemotherapy during the period of cranial irradiation (5–6 injections) and 33 out of 36 as a maintenance IT therapy (every 3 months) for 36–48 months; twenty-six children received IT MTX (6 mg/m^2 in 18 patients; 10 mg/m^2 in 8), total dose 36–160 mg/m^2 (medial 102); 13 patients received IT cytosine arabinoside (Ara-C) (6 mg/m^2), total dose 36–174 mg/m^2; 3 children received IT MTX plus ARA-C.

A control group consisting of 18 children with solid tumours off-therapy was also utilized for the neuropsychological study. Nine patients of this group were treated for Hodgkin's disease and 9 for Wilm's tumor.

These patients were aged 2.1–10 (median 4.8) years at diagnosis and 6.3–14 (median 9.2) years at this assessment. All patients were disease-free and off-therapy from 0.4 to 8.6 years (median 3.6 years). Each patient with ALL underwent CT brain scans, EEG and neuropsychological study. The CT brain scans were performed with EMI CT 1010 scanners with 10 mm collimation and a scan time of 60 seconds. In some patients contrast enhancement was employed.

EEG's were recorded utilizing the 10–20 system modified by Pampiglione (16). The investigation was performed mostly during the waking state; in addition photic stimulation and overbreathing were performed whenever possible.

Intellectual performance was measured by means of the Wechsler Intelligence Scale for Children (WISC); all the patients tested (those with ALL and those with solid tumours) were aged >6 years at the time of the study and had a comparable social background. Perceptual-motor ability was explored by means of the Bender

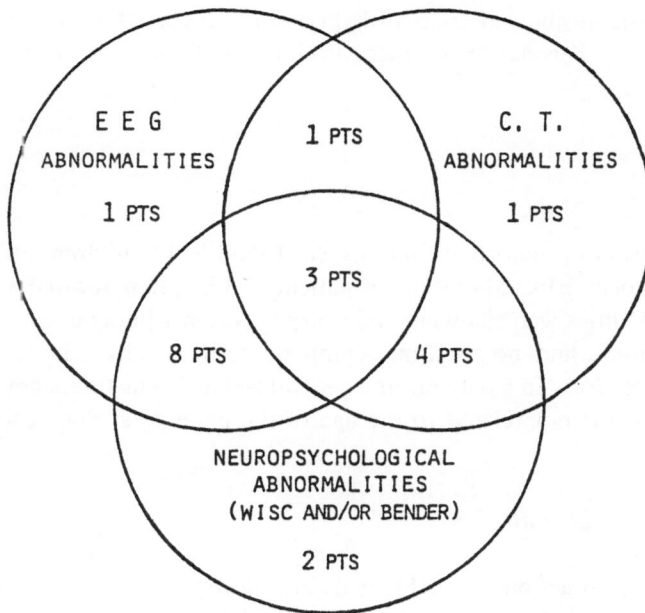

Figure 1. Correlations between CT brain scans, EEG and neuropsychological studies in 36 children with ALL off-therapy.
- 20/36 pts (55%) had one or more abnormalities:
- 12/21 (57%) pts aged <5 years at diagnosis
  8/15 (53%) pts aged ≥5 yeara at diagnosis

Visual Motor Gestalt test. Twenty children with ALL were re-tested after one year.

Leukemic children and children with tumours were compared on the WISC scores and the results of the Bender-Gestalt test. Children with ALL were grouped into two sub-groups for analysis, i.e. <5 and ≥5 years at the time of diagnosis, since it has been suggested that the age of the brain exposure to ionizing radiation might play an important role in the appearance of the brain injury (6, 7). CT brain scans, EEG and neuropsychological studies were compared of the two groups.

Results

CT brain scans

Abnormal findings were found in 9 out of 36 (25%) children with ALL. Intracerebral calcifications were present in 2 patients; ventricular dilatation in 3; subarachnoid space dilatation in 1; ventricular plus subarachnoid space dilatation in 1. Two patients showed areas of hypodensity in the white matter.

There was no correlation of these findings with the age of the patients at diagnosis.

EEG

A wide spectrum of abnormal findings was found in 13 children (36%). Slowing was the prevalent EEG alteration (6 patients); 3 children showed sharp waves; other abnormalities were: slowing and sharp waves in 1 patient; low amplitude in 1; low amplitude and no rhythmic components in 1; spikes in 1. These EEG alterations were focal in 6 patients and generalized in 7. The frequency of the EEG abnormalities was not related to the age of the patients at diagnosis.

Neuropsychological study

Mean scores obtained on the WISC scale in children with ALL and children with solid tumours showed a statistically significant difference between the two groups as far as verbal scale (P < 0.01) and full scale IQ (P < 0.01) are concerned, ALL children having the lowest scores, and children with solid tumours the highest (table 1).

A statistically significant difference between the two groups was also present in terms of numbers of patients with an abnormal Bender-Gestalt test (P < 0.01) Perceptual-motor disabilities were more frequent in ALL patients (17 of 36) than in the control group (2 of 18).

Twenty children with ALL were re-tested after a year and no statistically significant difference from the results of the first testing was found.

Table 1. Neuropsychological study comparison between children with ALL off-therapy and children with solid tumours off-therapy, of comparable age.

	N. pts	WISC (mean scores)			Bender-gestalt test	
		Verbal scale	Performance scale	Overall IQ	Normal n. pts	Abnormal n. pts
ALL off-therapy*	36	93.3	91.7	91.6	19	17
Solid tumours off-therapy	18	105.2	100	102.6	16	2
		p < 0.01	p < 0.05	p < 0.01	p < 0.01	

* No statistically significant difference was found in 20 pts retested after 1 year.

Table 2. Neuropsychological study comparison between ALL children aged <5 and ≥5 years at diagnosis.

	N. pts	WISC (mean scores)			Bender-gestalt test	
		Verbal scale	Performance scale	Overall IQ	Normal n. pts	Abnormal n. pts
ALL <5 years at diagnosis	21	95.1	95	94.1	8	13
ALL ≥5 years at diagnosis	15	90.6	87.2	88	11	4
		NS	NS	NS	$p < 0.05$	

When the ALL children were divided into two sub-groups according to age at diagnosis, no statistically significant difference in the WISC scale was found (Table 2). In contrast the Bender-Gestalt test was abnormal in 13 out of 21 children of the younger group, whereas it was abnormal only in 4 out of 11 of the older one.

Correlations between CT brain scans, EEG and neuropsychological studies

In figure 1 we have summarized patient distribution according to the presence of one or more abnormalities in CT, EEG and neuropsychological studies. Twenty out of the 36 ALL children (55%) had one or more abnormalities; 12 of these patients were aged <5 years and 8 patients >5 years at diagnosis. The incidence of CNS abnormalities was not related to the interval since cranial irradiation or to the drugs (MTX or Ara-C) used for IT therapy.

Clinical symptoms

Twelve out of 36 ALL children (33%) experienced the somnolence syndrome. Five of these patients had one or more CNS abnormalities. Three children aged 1.7, 2.3 and 9 years at the time of diagnosis presented with seizures at 1.5, 2 and 3 years following cranial irradiation. Two of these patients had intracerebral calcifications; one had ventricular and subarachnoid space widening.

Discussion

Four types of CT abnormalities have been noted in patients who have received

CNS prophylaxis: ventricular dilatation, areas of decreased attenuation coefficient (hypodense areas in white matter), intracerebral calcifications and subarachnoid space dilatation. These types of abnormalities have been mainly attributed to the combination of IT MTX, high dose IV MTX and cranial irradiation (13, 19, 20); IT MTX plus cranial irradiation also can produce CT scan changes (8, 18). A lower incidence of CT abnormalities has been noted with IT MTX alone or IT MTX plus high dose IV MTX without cranial irradiation (12, 15).

The frequency of CT abnormalities in our patients (25%) is less than in Peylan-Ramu's patients (53%) treated in a similar fashion (IT MTX or IT Ara-C plus cranial irradiation). This may be due to the greater intensity of IT chemotherapy in that study.

Few data on EEG abnormalities in children with ALL off-therapy are available. Freeman described diffuse slow wave distribution over both cerebral hemispheres in the post-irradiation somnolence syndrome (10). Pampiglione felt that a distinction should be made between a 'diffuse generalized abnormality' and 'focal' changes in which some regions of the brain are affected differently than others (17). Fassetta studied 24 ALL children and found EEG changes to be inconsistent over time (9). A detailed analysis of EEG's has been made by Ch'ien and coworkers (2) who studied 49 ALL children longitudinally. All 49 patients had abnormally slow EEG background frequencies during the four-year study, mainly during the period of the post-irradiation somnolence syndrome.

In our study we found no correlation between the somnolence syndrome and long-term neurological dysfunction as detected by EEG studies.

As others had described (5, 6, 7) we also noted intellectual impairment and perceptual-motor disabilities in our ALL patients. The differences pointed out in this study between the ALL patients and the control group (children with solid tumours) seem to suggest that CNS prophylaxis is a crucial problem in the treatment of ALL.

Surprisingly, no clear correlation between the frequency of CNS adverse sequelae and patient age at diagnosis (i.e. at the time of cranial irradiation) has been found in our study. Other investigators (6, 7) have stressed that the younger brain is more vulnerable to adverse effects of chemotherapy and irradiation than the mature brain.

An alternative hypothesis is the view that the injury to CNS in the child is less severe than the effects of comparable injury in the adult, because the developing organism is endowed with compensatory mechanisms which the adult lacks.

The high number of patients with one or more abnormalities might be related to the high total dose of IT MTX (>50 mg/m^2) administered as maintenance therapy. However, in contrast to the high incidence of subtle CNS impairment revealed by EEG and psychometric tests, overt clinical symptoms of CNS toxicity were present in only a few patients.

Our results suggest that prospective multidisciplinary studies are needed to determine the true incidence of CNS injury as a result of CNS prophylaxis. Such a study is in progress in our institution at the present time.

Acknowledgements

The authors are grateful to Dr. G. Missiroli (Institute of Psychology, University of Bologna), Dr. L. Sabattini (Department of Neuroradiology, 'Bellaria' Hospital, Bologna), Dr. E. Franzoni (Department of Pediatrics, EEG Service, University of Bologna) for their help. This study was supported by CNR, PFCCN N.81.01430.96.

References

1. Bleyer WA, Griffin TW: White Matter Necrosis, Mineralizing Microangiopathy, and Intelletual Abilities in Survivors of Childhood Leukemia. Associations with Central Nervous System Irradiation and Methotrexate Therapy. Radiation Damage to the Nervous System. Gilbert HA and Kagan AR (eds.), Raven Press, New York, pp. 155–277, 1980.
2. Ch'ien LT, Aur RJA, Verzosa MS, Coburn TP, Goff JR, Hustu HO, Price RA, Seifert MJ, Simone JV: Progression of Methotrexate-Induced Leukoencephalopathy in Children with leukemia. Med and Ped Oncol 9:133–141, 1981.
3. Ch'ien LT, Aur RJA, Stagner S, Cavallo K, Wood A, Goff J, Pitner S, Hustu HO, Seifert MJ, Simone JV: Long-Term Neurological Implications of Somnolence Syndrome in children with acute lymphocytic leukemia. Annals of Neurology 8:273–277, 1980.
4. Crosley CJ, Rorke LB, Evans A, Nigro M: Central nervous system lesions in childhood leukemia. Neurology 28:678–685, 1978.
5. Eiser C: Intellectual abilities among survivors of childhood leukemia as a function of CNS irradiation. Arch Dis Child 53:391–395, 1978.
6. Eiser C: Effects of chronic illness on intellectual development. Arch Dis Child 55:766–770, 1980.
7. Eiser C, Lansdown R: Retrospective study of intellectual development in children with acute lymphoblastic leukemia. Arch Dis Child 52:525–529, 1977.
8. Enzmann DR, Lane B: Enlargment of subarachnoid spaces and lateral ventricles in pediatric patients undergoing chemotherapy. J Pediat 92:535–539, 1978.
9. Fassetta G. Carli M, Cante G: EEG changes in leukemic children following cranial irradiation with Cobalt 60 associated with intrathecal chemotherapy. EEG and Clinical Neurophysiology 41:326–327, 1976 (abstract.
10. Freeman J, Johnston PG, Voke JM: Somnolence after prophylactic cranial irradiation in children with acute lymphoblastic leukemia in remission. Br Med J 5:523, 1979.
11. Kay HEM. Knapton IJ, O'Sullivan JZ, et al: Encephalopathy in acute leukaemia associated with methotrexate therapy. Arch Dis Child 47:344, 1972.
12. Kolmannskog S, Moe PJ, Anke IM: CT findings of the brain in children with acute lymphocytic leukemia after CNS prophylaxis without cranial irradiation. Acta Paed Scand 68:875, 1979.
13. McIntosh S, Fischer DB, Rothman SG, Rosenfield N, Label JS, O'Brien RT: Intracranial calcifications in childhood leukemia. J Pediat 91:909–913, 977.
14. Meadows AT, Evans AE: Effects of chemotherapy on the central nervous system. A study of parenteral methotrexate in long-term survivors of leukemia and lymphoma in childhood. Cancer 37 (Suppl) 1079–1985, 1976.

15. Ochs JS, Berger P, Brecher M, Sinks LF, Kinkel W, Freeman AI: Computed tomography scans in children with acute lymphocytic leukemia receiving methotrexate alone as Central Nervous System prophylaxis. Cancer 45:2274–2278, 1980.

16. Pampiglione G: Some anatomical considerations upon electrode placement in routine EEG. Proc Electrophysiol Techn Ass 7:20, 1956.

17. Pampiglione G: Somnolence in children with acute leukemia. Letter. British Med J. p 158, 26 June, 1974.

18. Peylan-Ramu N, Poplack DG, Pizzo PA, Adornato BT, DeChiro G: Abnormal CT scans of the brain in asymptomatic children with acute lymphocytic leukemia after prophylactic treatment of the central nervous system with radiation and intrathecal chemotherapy. NEJM 298:815–818, 1978.

19. Price RA, Birdwell DA: The central nervous system in childhood leukemia. III Mineralizing microangiopathy and dystrophic calcification. Cancer 42:717–728, 1978.

20. Price RA, Jamieson PA: The central nervous system in childhood leukemia. II. Subacute leukoencephalopthy. Cancer 35:306, 1975.

21. Rubinstein LJ, Herman MM, Lory TF, Wilbur JR: Disseminated necrotizing leukoencephalopathy. A complication of treated central nervous system leukemia and lymphoma. Cancer 35:291–305, 1975.

13. Treatment of Overt CNS Leukaemia

M.L.N. WILLOUGHBY

Introduction

The first MRC Meningeal Leukaemia Trial (1) showed that further CNS relapse developed in only 2 out of 9 children treated by the combined modality approach of intrathecal Methotrexate (IT MTX) to clear the CSF of blast cells followed by craniospinal radiotherapy. In those randomized to have cranial only, rather than craniospinal, radiotherapy there was no comparable benefit; 8 out of 8 developing further CNS relapse. These results were obtained in a group of children who had not received previous prophylactic CNS irradiation and who were being treated for their first isolated CNS relapse.

The present report concerns:

1. Long-term follow up of the original series of children treated by IT MTX and craniospinal irradiation for overt CNS leukaemia.
2. The question of whether this therapy can be used in previously irradiated children without either loss of efficacy or risk of encephalopathy.
3. Whether the addition of systemic reinduction or intensification can reduce the liability to marrow and testicular relapse after apparently isolated CNS relapse.
4. Possible alternative approaches to the treatment of overt CNS leukaemia currently being explored.

1. Eight-year follow up after treatment of isolated CNS relapse

The problem in treatment of CNS leukaemia is not that of obtaining a remission, which occurred in 35 of 36 children after IT MTX in the MRC trial (1), but of preventing subsequent CNS, systemic or extramedullary relapse.

Intrathecal drugs alone are unlikely to eradicate overt CNS leukaemia because perivascular cuffing (2) renders the deepest-placed cells inaccessible to drugs in the CSF (3). But by following a cyto-reductive course of IT MTX with whole CNS (craniospinal) irradiation we may fortuitously have taken advantage of the expected enhanced radiosensitivity of the smaller tumour cell burden (4) in these highly radiosensitive (5) cells. All patients received 2,500 rads to the cranium and half were randomized to an additional 1,000 rads given contemporaneously to the

R. Mastrangelo, D.G. Poplack, R. Riccardi (eds), Central Nervous System Leukemia. ISBN 978-94-009-6710-6.
© 1983 Martinus Nijhoff Publishers, Boston.

spine. The earlier report (1) that only 2 out of 9 in the craniospinal arm developed further CNS recurrence compared to 8 out of 8 in the cranial arm has remained true at 8-year follow up (Figure 1). Both CNS remission duration and disease-free survival (Figure 2) are significantly superior in the craniospinal arm of this prospectively randomized trial (Log rank analysis (6), P <0.001). Survival has been compromised more by the 5 instances of marrow relapse than by the 2 of further CNS relapse. The marrow relapses at 47 and 55 months (Figure 1) had shortly been preceded by testicular relapse. A similarly high incidence of systemic recurrence has been found after isolated CNS relapse in other series (7, 8). Nevertheless, 2 out of the 9 children on the craniospinal consolidation arm are disease-free survivors beyond 8 years from their CNS relapse and off all systemic therapy for 6 years.

A recent independent analysis (9) of a total of 57 children who developed isolated CNS relapse while on the early MRC trials and not given prophylactic CNS radiation has shown a similar advantage of craniospinal compared to cranial or no irradiation following IT MTX (Figure 3). This larger series includes the 17 cases randomized on the MRC meningeal trial in addition to others treated in a similar way in MRC centres but by physician preference rather than by randomization. 7 of 16 are surviving free of recurrence between 80 and 130 months after craniospinal compared to 1 (at 100 months) of 11 after cranial and none (beyond 20 months) of 30 after IT MTX alone (Log Rank Analysis, P <0.001).

It appears from these findings that isolated CNS relapse developing in previously unirradiated children can be effectively treated by craniospinal

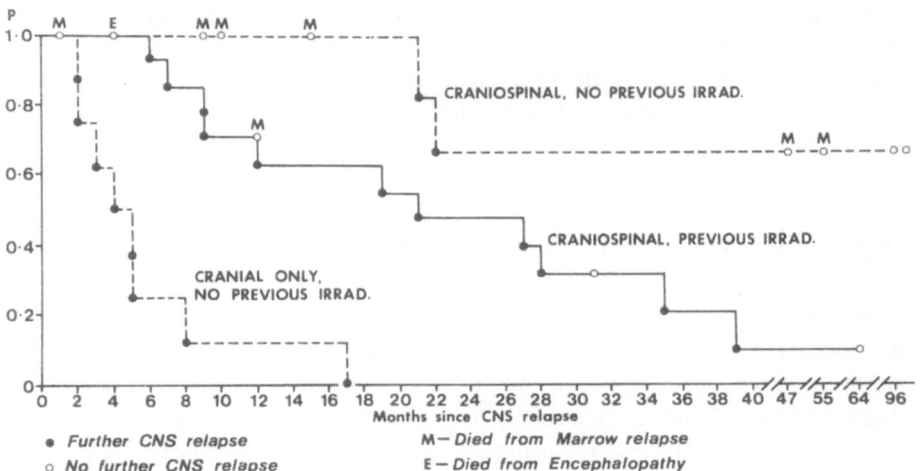

Figure 1. Follow-up of MRC Meningeal Leukaemia Trial (1) (dotted lines) with superimposed results from craniospinal schedule applied to a later series of previously-irradiated children developing CNS leukaemia.

Log Rank Analysis shows: p <0.01 for difference between upper 2 arms; p <0.001 for difference between lower 2 arms.

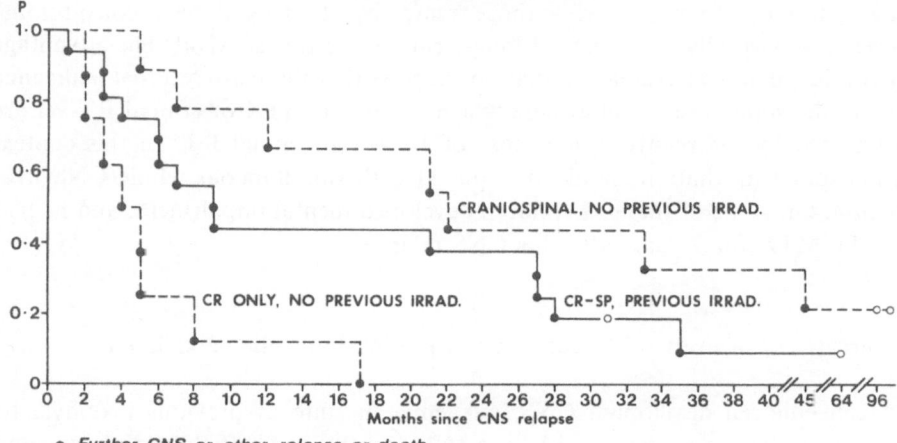

DISEASE-FREE SURVIVAL

Figure 2. Follow-up of same patients as in Figure 1, but showing disease-free survival.
$p < 0.05$ for upper 2 arms; $p < 0.001$ for lower 2 arms.

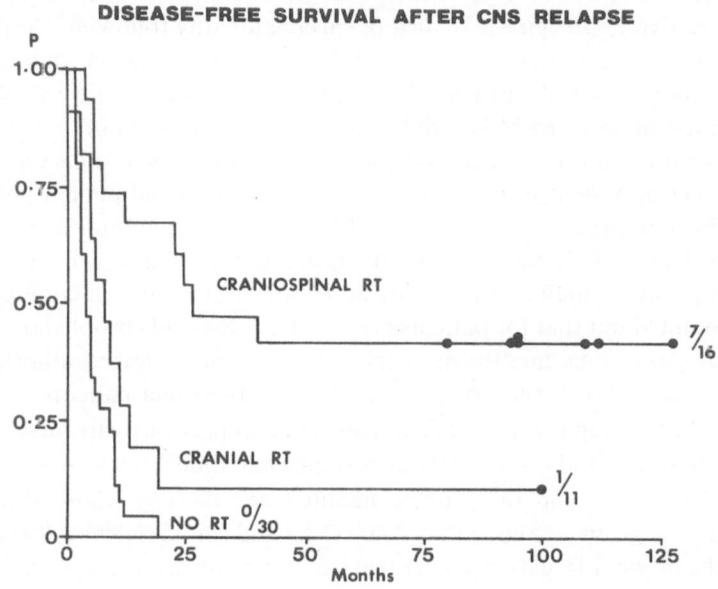

DISEASE-FREE SURVIVAL AFTER CNS RELAPSE

Figure 3. Patients developing CNS leukaemia on early MRC trials (Concord and UKALL I) not given prophylactic RT, and treated for CNS leukaemia in different ways.
$p < 0.01$ for upper 2 arms; $p < 0.001$ for lower 2 arms.

irradiation after CSF clearance by IT MTX with worthwhile long-term remission in 25% to 40% of patients, while those treated by IT MTX alone at conventional doses have virtually no chance of long-term disease-free survival. The advantage of craniospinal over cranial irradiation suggests that there are residual leukaemic foci in the spinal area or elsewhere which escape IT MTX or cranial RT yet are eradicated by the relatively low dose of 1,000 rads spinal RT. In this context craniospinal irradiation should be equated with simultaneous whole CNS irradiation. Only one of these 57 children developed mental impairment, and he had had IT MTX for 7 years after his CNS relapse.

2. Treatment of overt CNS leukaemia in previously irradiated children

Sixteen children developing CNS leukaemia in spite of previous prophylactic cranial irradiation were treated by the MRC centres in Sheffield, Edinburgh and Glasgow with the same schedule of IT MTX and craniospinal RT as in the earlier trial (1) to determine whether there would be either loss of efficacy or risk of encephalopathy when applied to such patients. The CNS remission and disease-free survival curves were significantly inferior to those obtained in previously unirradiated children, but still significantly superior to the earlier control (cranial only) arm (Figures 1 and 2). Two of the 16 are surviving without further recurrence $2\frac{1}{2}$ and 5 years after their CNS relapse, off all therapy 1 and 3 years respectively. One girl of 16 died of encephalopathy following Herpes Zoster but to which intraventricular MTX (via Ommaya reservoir) and repeat RT probably contributed. A further 17 children have been treated by similar repeat CNS irradiation in a 3rd MRC trial (Figure 4, Table 1) without any instances of encephalopathy, but a criterion for entry to this trial was an *interval of at least 6 months between the two courses of cranial RT*. A non-trial patient given repeat RT within 6 months of prophylactic 2,400 rads to the cranium developed fatal encephalopathy. With the precaution of this 6-month interval the hazard of encephalopathy is small and probably acceptable in the clinical context. Jenkins (10) has pointed out that for patients given initial 1,800 rads prophylaxis a further 2,400 rads given some months or years later represents a lesser radiotherapeutic dose than the 3,500–4,000 rads given to Medulloblastoma patients.

The St. Jude group (7) treated CNS leukaemia in previously irradiated patients (2,400 rads from Study V or VII) in a somewhat similar way. After IT MTX, continued until the end of systemic maintenance therapy, those still in CNS remission were given cranial (2,000–2,400 rads) and spinal (1,500–2,000 rads) RT. Four of the original 16 patients remained free of any recurrence at over 30 months from their CNS relapse (Table 1).

The 5% to 10% of patients who develop CNS relapse in spite of contemporary forms of CNS prophylaxis may represent a self-selected group with more aggressive disease reflected by their greater liability to CNS and systemic relapse.

MRC MENINGEAL LEUKAEMIA STUDY III

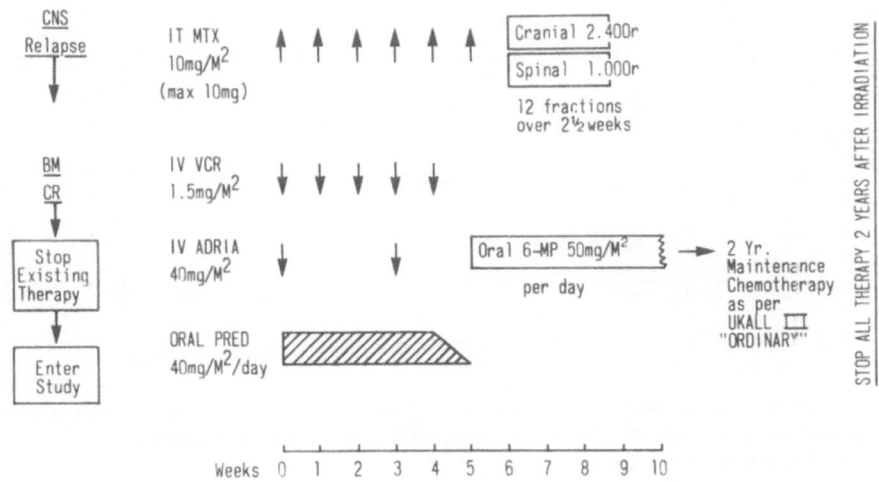

Figure 4. Diagram of protocol for 3rd MRC Meningeal Leukaemia Study.

Table 1. Disease-free survival after CNS leukemia in previously irradiated children.

Study	Therapy after CNS leukaemia	Total number	Number in complete remission	Duration
MRC	IT MTX, craniospinal radiotherapy maintenance 2 years	16*	2	2½ and 5 years
St. Jude (3)	IT MTX, maintenance, craniospinal radiotherapy	16	4	at 30 mo.
Indianapolis (11)	IT MTX, IV vincristine, L-asparaginase, prednisone, craniospinal radiotherapy, maintenance	10	5	13 to 37 mo.
MRC III	IT MTX, IV vincristine, adriamycin, prednisone, craniospinal radiotherapy, maintenance	17	6	8 to 26 mo.
Totals		59	17 (28.8%)	

* 1 case of encephalopathy.

118

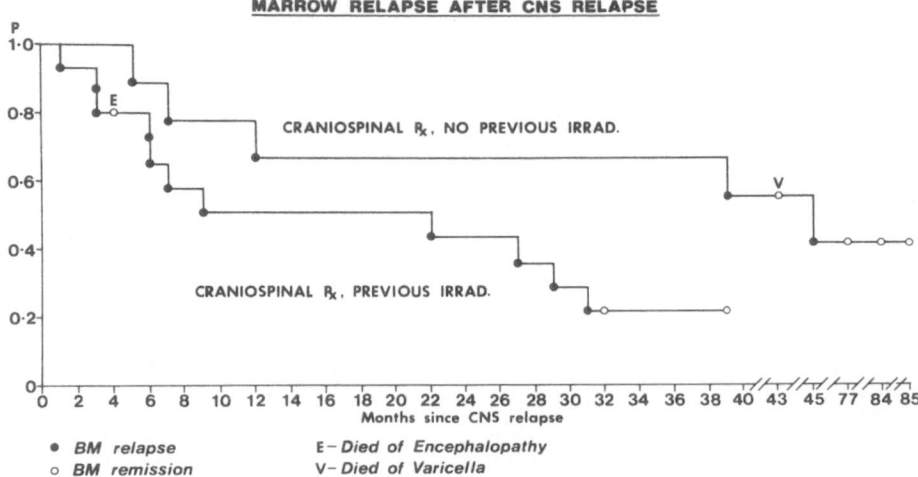

Figure 5. Comparison of incidence of marrow relapse after isolated CNS relapse in children with or without previous prophylactic CNS RT. (All treated in same way for CNS relapse). p<0.01 (Long Rank Analysis).

This was not necessarily true of the 50% or so who developed CNS relapse without prophylaxis. This is supported by the higher cumulative incidence of marrow relapse in the two MRC studies of CNS leukaemia in previously irradiated children than in the earlier trial in unirradiated children (Figure 5). The same conclusion was reached from analysis (11) of the American CCSG Study 101 which stated that 'the frequency of subsequent marrow relapse after isolated CNS relapse is not as high as in patients whose disease breaks through after receiving adequate CNS prophylaxis'. Standard therapy may therefore be inadequate for the group of patients currently being encountered who develop CNS leukaemia in spite of previous irradiation, and more intensive systemic therapy, in addition to the CNS therapy, may be needed if any are to be salvaged.

3. Reinduction and intensified systemic therapy in addition to CNS therapy

The high incidence of systemic relapse in those whose CNS leukaemia had been well controlled by craniospinal RT (Figure 1) in the first MRC trial, and the fact that all but one of the 2nd CNS relapses in the 2nd trial had been preceded by an intervening systemic relapse, led to the design of the 3rd MRC protocol for CNS leukaemia (Figure 4). This employed Vincristine, Adriamycin and Prednisolone systemic reinduction during the course of IT MTX preceding craniospinal RT, and was followed by a further 2 years of maintenance systemic therapy. Intramuscular L-Asparaginase could with advantage have been added to the reinduction phase (6,000 units/m^2 × 3 per week for 9 doses) as is employed in a current American protocol (12). The need for additional systemic chemotherapy at times of CNS relapse is justified also by the concepts (1) that 'isolated' CNS relapse is not always totally isolated, and (2) that those developing CNS relapse in spite of earlier prophylaxis have a more aggressive form of leukaemia.

At the present time the CNS remission and disease-free survival curves of patients entered on the 3rd MRC study (Figure 4) are closely following those of the earlier study for previously irradiated patients with 6 out of 20 free of recurrence at 8 to 26 months, and with the benefit of this form of reinduction not yet proven. Encouraging results, however, have been reported by Baehner and co-workers (12) in Indianapolis in children with CNS relapse after CCSG protocols using 1,800 or 2,400 rads cranial prophylaxis. They gave 6 bi-weekly doses of IT MTX followed by 2,400 rads cranial plus 1,200 rads spinal RT, followed by a further 12 doses of IT MTX spread over 18 months. IV Vincristine, oral Prednisolone and IM L-Asparaginase were given as systemic reinduction. Of 10 with primary isolated CNS relapse 5 developed a marrow relapse, CNS recurrence or other neurological sequelae within 7 months, but the remaining 5 have continued in remission for 13 to 37 months after their CNS relapse. It is possible that even more intensive systemic therapy such as intermediate-dose MTX infusions should be considered in future studies. The present results from MRC, St. Jude (7) and Indianapolis (12) studies in previously irradiated patients are given in Table 1, and indicate that repeat CNS irradiation after IT MTX is an acceptable approach without frequent serious CNS toxicity and with a total of 12 out of 59 (28%) currently surviving free of further recurrence.

Further support for the value of systemic reinduction (Vincristine plus Prednisolone) at the time of CNS relapse comes from a retrospective analysis (9) of the same cases as shown in Figure 3, from early MRC trials and not given CNS prophylaxis. A significantly improved disease-free survival at 75 to 125 months occurred in those given such reinduction compared to those who did not in this non-randomized cohort of patients (Figure 6).

4. New and experimental approaches to treatment of CNS leukaemia

Alternative and experimental approaches include the surgical insertion of an Ommaya reservoir for purposes of direct intraventricular installation of MTX since this route results in more dependable ventricular CSF drug levels (13) and avoids the discomfort of repeated lumbar punctures. The Memorial Sloan Kettering group have employed subcutaneous Ommaya reservoirs for maintenance CNS chemotherapy after initial clearance of CSF blast cells by intralumbar MTX and ARA-C.

Of 10 children treated for overt CNS leukaemia 3 showed CNS recurrence, one with simultaneous testicular followed by BM relapse. Another had an early BM relapse and 6 remain in CNS remission at 12–62 months, three being off chemotherapy for 1, 2 and 26 months. Median duration of CNS remission was approximately 30 months which is comparable to the results of the MRC trial. These results are impressive, especially as the schedule avoids the possible hazards of RT. Yet intraventricular chemotherapy should have the same limitation as was stated for IT chemotherapy in curative potential viz. that the deep perivascular 'cuffing' seen in advanced CNS leukaemia should preclude access of drugs in the subarachnoid space reaching the most deeply placed cells (3).

Bleyer & Poplack (14) utilized the Ommaya reservoir technique to explore an experimental pharmacokinetic approach to the treatment of CNS leukaemia. By giving 1 mg MTX every 12 hours for 6 doses the CSF level remained at a cytocidal level ($> 10^{-6}$ M) for 72 hours encompassing the S-phase of the leukaemic cell cycle. By contrast a single injection of 12 mg/m^2 maintained this therapeutic level for less than 32 hours. This approach also reduced the high peak CSF MTX level thought to be contributory to MTX neurotoxicity (15). Clinical results showed that the repeated smaller doses ('C × T regimen') were equally effective but less neurotoxic, and reduced the cumulative MTX dose by 50%.

A further extension of the use of the Ommaya reservoir is ventriculo-lumbar cerebrospinal perfusion for treatment of refractory meningeal leukaemia (14). This is a complex procedure reserved for patients resistant to normal therapy. MTX is administered into the ventricular CSF and perfused throughout the CSF, being finally removed via an outflow cannula in the lumbar subarachnoid space. CSF pressure in controlled by the height of the outflow column. By this technique high concentrations of MTX can be delivered to the whole subarachnoid space, including the cerebral convexities. Clinical and cytological remission was obtained after 4-hour infusion of 5×10^{-4} Molar MTX in a patient who was previously refractory to IT MTX, IT ARA-C, IT Hydroxyurea, IT Hydrocortisone and finally 'C × T' ventricular MTX (17).

In a review of 'Experimental Approaches to the Treatment of CNS Leukaemia' Poplack, Bleyer and Pizzo (17) mention also the pharamacological fact that IV infusions of MTX (600 mg/m^2 for 1 hour and 120 mg/m^2 per hour for 41 hours) achieve a cytocidal lumbar and ventricular CSF concentrations of MTX (greater than 10^{-6} M) for the duration of the infusion. This would have the same theoretical advantages as the 'C × T' Ommaya approach but without recourse to surgical intervention and with the added advantage that it should provide entrance of drug at all levels of the cerebrospinal axis and might reach systemic sanctuary sites as well, but it has yet to be tested clinically. These are the same considerations that led the Roswell Park group to use IV MTX infusions as CNS prophylaxis (18) as described earlier. Concepts developed for CNS therapy, whether preventive or for overt disease are to some extent interchangeable.

Looking ahead, and bearing in mind the propensity to systemic relapse after CNS leukaemia viz. the systemic nature of this complication, we are exploring the efficacy of total body irradiation and bone marrow transplantation, following the

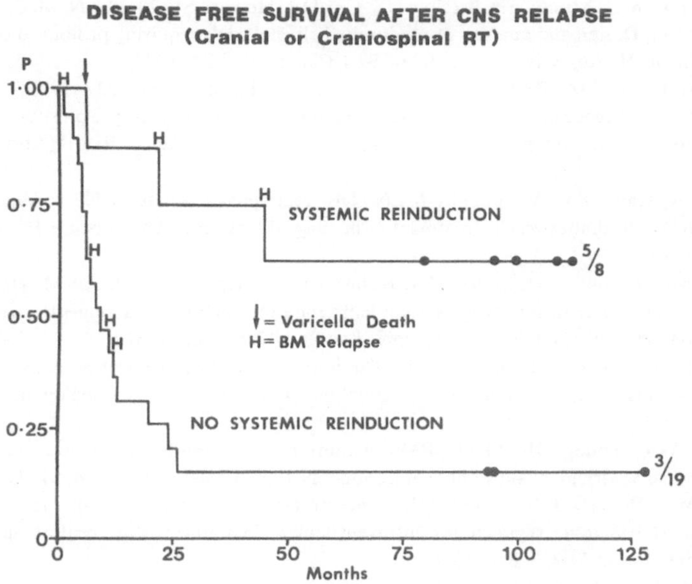

DISEASE FREE SURVIVAL AFTER CNS RELAPSE
(Cranial or Craniospinal RT)

Figure 6. Effect of systemic reinduction at time of CNS relapse on subsequent disease-free survival. Same children as in Figure 3 but excluding those treated by IT MTX alone. p < 0.01 (Log Rank Analysis).

current Seattle Schedule with additional IT MTX (19), in children brought back to total remission by IT MTX after isolated CNS relapse. Of 4 patients treated this way at the Royal Hospital for Sick Children in Glasgow, one, who had suffered two CNS relapses and had received two previous episodes of CNS RT 3 and 6 years earlier, is surviving without recurrence 1 year post-transplant. Three, however, died of transplant complications (Pneumonitis, GVHD, nutritional problems) at 3, 4 and 9 months post-transplant without evidence of CNS or systemic leukaemia but emphasizing the hazards of this approach.

References

1. Willoughby MLN: Treatment of overt meningeal leukaemia in children: results of second MRC meningeal leukaemia trial. Br Med J:864–867, 1976.
2. Price RA, Johnson WW: The central nervous system in childhood leukemia. I. The arachnoid. Cancer 31:520–533, 1973.
3. Price RA: Histopathology of CNS leukemia and complications of therapy. Am J Pediatr Hematol Oncol 1:21–30, 1979.
4. Moss WT, Brand WN, Battifora H: Radiation oncology; Rationale, Technique, Results. (ed 4). Saint Louis. C.V. Mosby Co. 1973, p. 22.
5. Cook JC, Considine B: Low-dose radiation therapy for leukemic involvement of the central nervous system. Radiology 104:649–652, 1972.

6. Peto R, Pike MC, Armitage P, Breslow NE, Cox DR, Howard SV, Mantel N, McPherson K, Peto J, Smith PG: Design and analysis of randomised clinical trials requiring prolonged observation of each patient. II. Analysis and examples. Br J Cancer 35:1–39, 1977.
7. Hustu HO, Aur RJA: Extramedullary leukemia. Clin Haemat 7:313–337, 1978.
8. Nesbit ME: Influence of an isolated central nervous system (CNS) relapse on subsequent marrow relapse in childhood lymphoblastic leukemia. Proc Am Assoc Cancer Res 18(Abstract 569):143, 1977.
9. Rankin A, Kay HEM, Willoughby MLN: The treatment of isolated CNS leukaemia. In press.
10. Jenkin RDT: Radiation in the treatment of meningeal leukemia. Am J Pediatr Hematol Oncol 1: 49–58, 1979.
11. Nesbit ME, D'Angio GJ, Sather HN, Robison LL, Ortega J, Donaldson M, Hammond GD: Effect of isolated central nervous system leukaemia on bone marrow remission and survival in childhood acute lymphoblastic leukaemia. Lancet 1:1386–1388, 1981.
12. Wells RJ, Weetman RM, Baehner RL: The impact of isolated central nervous system relapse following initial complete remission in childhood acute lymphoblastic leukemia. J Pediatr 97: 429–432, 1980.
13. Shapiro WR, Young DF, Mehta BM: Methotrexate distribution in cerebrospinal fluid after intravenous, ventricular and lumbar injections. N Engl J Med 293:161–166, 1975.
14. Bleyer WA, Poplack DG, Simon RH: Concentration × time methotrexate via a subcutaneous reservoir: a less toxic regimen for intraventricular chemotherapy of central nervous system neoplasms. Blood 51:835–842, 1978.
15. Pizzo PA, Poplack DG, Bleyer WA: Neurotoxicities of current leukemia therapy. Am J Pediatr Hematol Oncol 1:127–140, 1979.
16. Rubin RC, Ommaya AK, Henderson ES et al: Cerebrospinal fluid perfusion for central nervous system neoplasms. Neurology 16:680–692, 1966.
17. Poplack DG, Bleyer WA, Pizzo PA: Experimental approaches to the treatment of CNS leukemia. Am J Pediatr Hemat Oncol 1:141–149, 1979.
18. Freeman AI, Wang JJ, Sinks LF: High dose methotrexate in acute lymphocytic leukemia. Cancer Treat Rep 61:727–731, 1977.
19. Thomas Ed, Buckner CD, Clift TA et al: Marrow transplantation for acute nonlymphoblastic leukemia in first remission. N Engl J Med 301:597–599, 1979.

14. Radiation Therapy Methods for the Treatment of Central Nervous System Leukemia

A. OAKHILL and G.J. D'ANGIO

It has long been known that radiation therapy can relieve the symptoms and signs of meningeal leukemia. Decades ago, remissions were short lived when low doses (e.g., about 450 rad) were employed; in any case, survival was poor because of high bone marrow relapse rates (1). This discussion will concentrate on the therapy of CNS leukemia in the modern era of successful chemotherapy for acute leukemia in childhood.

Several radiation therapy (RT) methods have been used for the treatment of meningeal leukemia once it becomes manifest. These have included cranial irradiation with or without a spinal component and given in a single course or in pulses (1, 2). Irradiation has been combined with intrathecal chemotherapy given via the lumbar route or intraventricularly (Ommaya device), instillation of radioactive colloids through a lumbar puncture, and combinations of these several methods (3, 4).

Years ago, patients with overt signs and symptoms of CNS leukemia were given low doses of radiation therapy (400 rad) directed to the symptomatic area. The response rate was 98% for 500 episodes of CNS disease managed in this way, and the mean symptom-free interval was 11 weeks (5).

The Children's Cancer Study group conducted a study (CCG-101) in which different systems of central nervous system 'prophylaxis' were employed. Patients were divided among four groups; Group 1 children received 2400 rad craniospinal irradiation (RT) plus 1200 rad to an extended field to include the liver, spleen, kidneys and gonads. Group 2 received 2400 rad to the craniospinal axis. Group 3 had 2400 rad to the cranium plus intrathecal methotrexate (IT MTX) 12 mg/sq. m. twice a week for three weeks, and Group 4 received IT MTX alone in doses similar to Group 3. Attention here will be directed only to patient Groups, 1, 2, and 3 who developed CNS relapse as a primary isolated event, as reported by Nesbit et al. (6). There were 20 such children among 318 with initial white blood cell counts under 20,000 per mm^3, and 11 among 128 with white blood cell counts greater than that number. Group 1 and 2 children who developed CNS relapse were treated with IT MTX twice weekly (12 mg/m^2) until the cerebro-spinal fluid (CSF) cleared. They then continued maintenance chemotherapy as it was given in that study along with IT MTX (12 mg/m^2) every month for 6 months. Regimen 3 children were treated differently; they were given 2400 rad to the cranio-spinal axis after which

R. Mastrangelo, D.G. Poplack, R. Riccardi (eds), Central Nervous System Leukemia. ISBN 978-94-009-6710-6.
© *1983 Martinus Nijhoff Publishers, Boston.*

maintenance chemotherapy resumed along with IT MTX monthly for six months. It is thus possible to compare the results of two different systems of 'salvage' therapy, one including radiation and the other not, in patients who had had identical induction and maintenance chemotherapy regimens and equally effective though different systems of prior CNS 'prophylaxis' at the time of consolidation. There was no obvious difference in the CNS outcome between the two systems of retrieval therapy. Five of the 20 with low initial counts suffered one or more additional CNS episodes, as did 5 of 11 with high counts. (Two of the latter developed concurrent bone marrow relapses.) All 3 of the 31 who survived free of any untoward event had low initial counts. It should be noted that the diagnosis of CNS relapse in CCG-101 was made when overt neurological signs became evident, not on the basis of routine lumbar punctures in asymptomatic patients.

Cook, Considine and their colleagues in Detroit used a different from of therapy. They have employed single courses of radiation therapy to the cranium, or the cranio-spinal axis after a one-week course of IT MTX. The doses used did not exceed about 160 rad delivered over two days. These courses were repeated as necessary when multiple episodes of CNS leukemia developed in any patient.

Their experience encompasses 143 consecutive children who received from 1 to 16 courses of combined IT MTX and RT. Four hundred twenty-three courses were delivered to the 143 children; 232 to the cranium alone, and 191 to the CNS axis. Ninety-seven percent of patients receiving cranio-spinal RT experienced relief of symptoms and signs vs. 87% for those given cranial irradiation alone. The median remission times, however, were 13 weeks for both groups, similar to that obtained by Evans et al. (5). Cook and colleagues report as their longest survivor a boy who was alive seven years after the diagnosis of leukemia and 164 weeks from the time meningeal leukemia was discovered. Sixteen courses of therapy were administered over the three-year interval. These data can be compared to the results in CCG-101/Regimen 4 children who received 'prophylactic' IT MTX in amounts now known to be inadequate for CNS prophylaxis (12 mg/m^2 2 × /wk × 3 wks). They are in this way roughly comparable to the patients reported by Cook et al., who had received no prior CNS 'prophylaxis'. The 55 CCG-101/ Regimen 4 patients with meningeal leukemia were treated in the same way as the relapsing regimen 3 children described above. The CNS control rate for the CCG children was 62%, a better result than that achieved by Evans et al. or the Detroit investigators.

In the second MRC meningeal leukemia trial, two groups of patients in their first meningeal relapse were compared (8). None of the patients studied had received prophylactic therapy. All patients received weekly intrathecal methotrexate until the CSF nucleated cell count was less than 10/mm^3 on two successive weeks. Patients were then randomized to receive cranial irradiation alone (8 patients) or craniospinal irradiation (9 patients). All of the children in the first group had a meningeal recurrence (median remission length 15 weeks) compared with only 2 in the second group (median remission length 99 weeks). Four children given craniospinal irradiation were alive 2.5 to 4 years after treatment for relapse.

Wells *et al.* reported their experience with ten children who had isolated CNS relapses after treatment according to standard CCG protocols (9). Patients who developed meningeal leukemia were given 2400 rad to the cranium, and 1200 rad to the spine after IT MTX (12 mg/m^2) twice a week until the CSF was clear and then once a week for six weeks. Eight of the ten patients then were given IT MTX every month for six months and then every other month for a year. Nine of the ten children also received reinduction chemotherapy (vincristine, prednisone, and L-asparaginase) for one month. This regimen resulted in a 27 month median relapse-free survival time; that is, without bone marrow, CNS, or other relapse. Only one of their patients developed recurrent meningeal leukemia, 6 and 11 months after the first CNS relapse. However, two others developed CNS signs, one leading to a fatal leukocencephalopathy, and a third child also has brain damage, possibly iatrogenic in origin. These results are to be compared with those reported by Willoughby (8), and by Hustu and Aur (10). The latter reported 16 patients who relapsed after 'prophylactic' radiation and who they attempted to treat with intrathecal methotrexate and continuation of maintenance chemotherapy, planning craniospinal radiation at the end of maintenance treatment. Unfortunately, 12 patients relapsed before this was possible (8 marrow, 4 second CNS) and thus only 8 children had retreatment of the CNS. At the time of the report there were 4 patients in continuous remission at 31 to 74 months.

The records of the Children's Hospital of Philadelphia from 1970 to 1979 were reviewed in this connection. There were five children with CNS leukemia at diagnosis; they are excluded from further consideration here. Twenty-three of 324 children, most of them treated according to CCSG protocols, developed CNS leukemia (7%). Retrieval was according to CCSG methods described above. Eight of the 23 had received no CNS 'prophylaxis'. Two of the eight children without CNS prophylaxis are alive after IT MTX and craniospinal irradiation of 2400 rad. Five of the six children who died in this group had white counts greater than 50,000/mm^3 and relapsed in the marrow at a median time of 5 months from diagnosis. These children survived for a median time of only 12 months after meningeal relapse.

Five of fifteen children who developed CNS relapse despite 'protection' are alive. These children were in remission longer than those who died (32 months vs 20 months) and the mean white count was lower (24×10^3/mm^3 vs 102×10^3/mm^3). Twelve of the 15 were re-induced using CCSG standard therapies (6), and 3 were given IT MTX alone. Four of the 12 in the former group are alive 9, 15, 30 and 50 months after re-treatment. All 3 who had only IT MTX suffered bone marrow relapses; only one is still alive 44 months after 4 additional CNS episodes and 2 bone marrow failures.

Overal survival for the 23 with meningeal leukemia was 30% and thus similar to the broader CCSG experience (6). Survival times in the children who died ranged from 7 to 53 months (median 22 months).

Investigators at Memorial Sloan-Kettering Cancer Center used a more complex system (3). Intralumbar methotrexate (MTX) (7 mg/m²) alternating with cytosine arabinoside (ARA-C) (25 mg/m²) was given preliminarily to relieve symptoms, an Ommaya reservoir was introduced, and this was followed with 600 rad to the craniospinal axis. Intraventricular MTX (7 mg/m²) was then given in two doses every 8 weeks over a period of three years. Their initial results were encouraging with an actuarially estimated 50% CNS relapse-free survival at three years in a group of 10 patients.

Paolucci and his colleagues in Bologna have used pulsed cranio-spinal irradiation in four patients who relapsed after prior irradiation and intrathecal chemotherapy. Six hundred to 1200 rad to a cranio-spinal field was given followed by 100 to 120 rad pulses every six weeks to four months plus intrathecal MTX with or without ARA-C. Three of the four patients developed CNS relapses with or without bone marrow relapses at 6, 7, and 13 months after initiation of this form of therapy; the other child relapsed in the bone marrow 20 months after therapy (11).

Sackmann-Muriel and his colleagues used radioactive colloidal phosphorous (RP) in a group of 16 patients who had suffered CNS relapse (12). Intrathecal MTX and dexamethasone was given first, and this was followed by three mCi of RP every six weeks. The CSF cleared for a median time of 360 days. However, the cauda equina syndrome (CES) developed in three patients. Zanesco and Carli also have employed RP in 11 patients with CNS relapse (13). Eight had acute leukemia and three had non-Hodgkin's lymphoma. All had received prior RT with or without IT MTX with or without ARA-C. One and one-half mCi of RP led to prompt clearing for a median time of 60 days (7).

Metz and Stoll reported their results in 10 patients who had 11 episodes of CNS leukemia among them. One of three mCi of 198-Au was given once and cleared the CSF in 8. They advocate external beam radiation therapy to follow. One of their patients developed the cauda equina syndrome (4). Earlier experience with 198-Au was less encouraging (14). Nine children with meningeal leukemialymphoma derived no prolonged benefit from the procedure (15).

Comment

It might be useful at this point to review the pathology of central nervous system leukemia when it is overt. Figure 1 shows the extensive perivascular cuffing with leukemia cells deep within the spinal cord that effectively prevents the penetration of any substance introduced into the subarachnoid space. Similar changes can be seen in the brain. These observations suggest that treatment plans should include the early use of external beam irradiation to lyse these deep-lying cells and thus open the pathways for the circulation of intrathecal medications. The system used at Memorial Hospital incorporates this notion, and it will be of interest to learn the

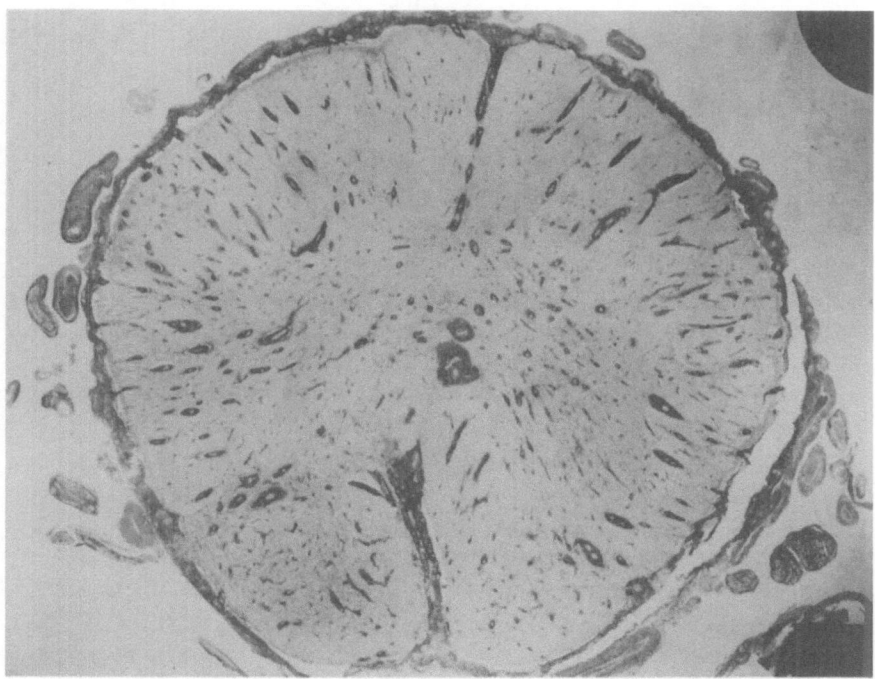

Figure 1. Cross section of spinal cord. There is meningeal infiltration and perviscular cuffing by leukemic cells. These latter changes are visible deep within the substance of the cord. Leukemic cells also infiltate among the fasciluli of the spinal nerve roots.

long-term follow-up in patients being managed that way.

An alternative method under study at the Children's Hospital of Philadelphia, collaborating with other investigators, is the periodic administration of external beam radiation plus IT MTX after an initial 'loading dose' of 450 rad in one session to the cranio-spinal axis. Monthly courses of 100 rad to the brain and spinal cord precede the administration of IT MTX.

It may be that the cells that repopulate the meninges after CNS 'prophylaxis' are less radio-responsive than the original population. The experience with children who develop CNS relapse after 'protection' tends to substantiate this. For example, 5 additional CNS relapses occurred in the 17 CCG-101/Regimen 3 patients who were given 2400 rad craniospinal irradiation at the time of the first meningeal leukemic episode. This might be because a different clone of cells survives the initial therapy, or the cells become resistant after repeated treatment, or a more resistant clone of cells survives systemic therapy. The latter contention is supported by the observation that 9 of 55 CCG-101/Regimen 4 children who first relapsed in the CNS developed repeated episodes of meningeal leukemia despite 2400 rad to the CNS given therapeutically. This rate (9/55 or 16%) is higher than

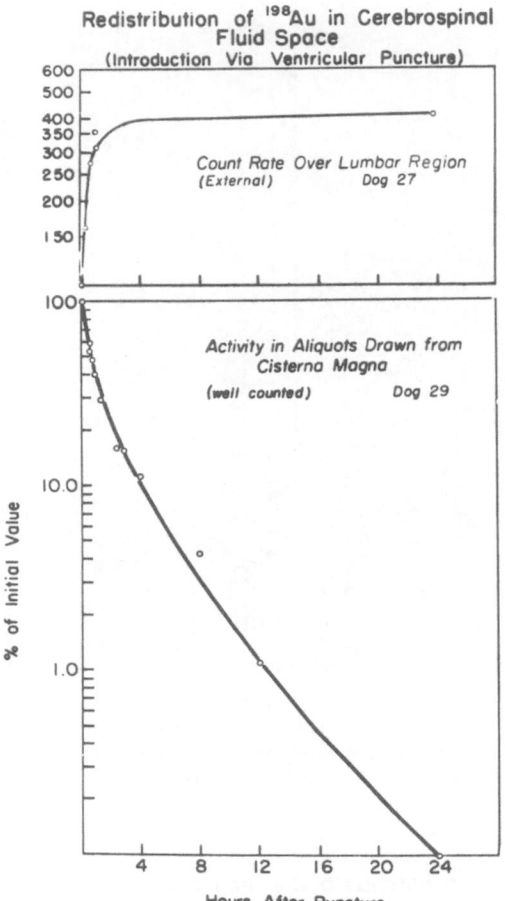

Figure 2. Laboratory study using a large-breed dog. The upper panel shows the rapid flow of radio-gold (RG) from the head to the tail when the animal was placed tail-down after RG was instilled via an intraventricular catheter.

The bottom panel shows the rapid disappearance of RG grom the cerebrospinal fluid due to ingestion of the colloid by parietal cells. (Figure reproduced from Kieffer SA, Stadlan EM, and D'Angio GJ: Acta Radiol 8:27–37, 1969, through the courtesy of Acta Radiologica.)

the overall CNS relapse rate in adequately protected CCSG patients (31/446 or 7%). It therefore would appear that higher doses of radiation are needed in order to control such patients. On the other hand, the major problem in children who develop meningeal leukemia after CNS 'prophylaxis' is bone marrow relapse. At least 65% of the 'protected' CCG-101 patients went on to develop bone marrow relapse within four years of the first episode of meningeal leukemia. Therefore, any system of therapy directed to leukemia in the brain and spinal cord must not jeopardize systemic chemotherapy. Moreover, many of these children will already have received cranial irradiation in doses of 1800 rad or more. Repeating that dose, especially in combination with methotrexate administered intrathecally, systemically, or both is associated with a relatively high frequency of leuko-encaphalopathy with its attendant adversities. The use of intrathecal radioactive colloids (RC) is attractive in this connection. Using suitable techniques, the RC can be made to distribute promptly and fairly evenly over the meningeal surfaces and recesses, where the major portion of the irradiation dose is delivered (Figure 2).

The bases of therapy most likely to provide the proper balance between control of CNS leukemia without compromising bone marrow reserve should probably include: 1. Lysis of anay perivascular leukemic infiltrate using external beam radiation therapy. Memorial Hospital has used 600 rad for this purpose. 2. Intermittent, relatively frequent administration of intrathecal (or intra-ventricular) medications with or without supplementary doses of external beam irradiation. If the latter are used, they are better given shortly before the intrathecal medicaments; e.g., one or two days. The agents to use intrathecally could include well-established single or multiple-drug regimens (e.g., metho-trexate, cytosine arabinoside, and hydrocortisone) or radioactive colloids such as radio-gold or radio-phosphorus.

Either of these methods should produce the least amount of bone marrow suppression, thus allowing energetic systemic re-induction and maintenance drugs to be administered.

A word of caution regarding the intrathecal administration of radioactive colloids: steps should be taken by appropriate preliminary studies to confirm that free flow of the material throughout the subarachnoid space can take place. Positioning to insure rapid distribution of the RC also is important (14). Caution should also be exercised when repeated doses of the agents are used because severe vascular and neurological damage can ensue (14).

References

1. Maurer AM: Therapy of acute lymphoblastic leukemia in childhood. Blood 56:1–10, 1980.
2. Considine B Jr, Cook JJ, Zuelzer WW, Ravindranath Y, Lusher JM: Repetitive low-dose radiation therapy for acute stem-cell leukemia. Int J Rad Onc Biol Phys 2:257–260, 1977.
3. Haghbin M, Galicich JH: Use of the Ommaya reservoir in the prevention and treatment of CNS leukemia. Amer J Pediatr Hematol/Oncol 1:111–117, 1979.
4. Metz O: Personal communication.
5. Evans AE, D'Angio GJ, Mitus A: Central nervous system complications of children with acute leukemia. J Ped 64:94–96, 1964.
6. Nesbit ME, Sather HN, Ortega J, D'Angio GJ, Robison LL, Donaldson M, Hammond GD: Effect of isolated central nervous system leukaemia on bone marrow remission and survival in childhood acute lymphoblastic leukaemia. Lancet i:1386–1389, 1981.
7. Cook JC, Considine B, Jr: Low-dose radiation therapy for leukemic involvement of the central nervous system. Radiology 104:649–652, 1972.

8. Willoughby MLN: Treatment of overt meningeal leukaemia in children: results of second MRC Meningeal Leukaemia Trial. Br Med J 1:864–867, 1976.
9. Wells RJ, Weetman RM, Baehner RL: The impact of isolated CNS relapse following initial complete remission in childhood acute lymphoblastic leukaemia. J Peds 97:3 429–432, 1980.
10. Hustu HO, Aur RJA: Extramedullary leukaemia. Clin Haematol 7:313, 1978.
11. Paolucci G: Personal communication.
12. Sackmann-Muriel F, Schere D, Barengols A, Eppinger-Helft M, Braier JF, Pavlovsky S, Macchi GH, Guman L: Remission maintenance therapy for meningeal leukaemia: Intrathecal methotrexate and dexamenthasone versus intrathecal craniospinal irradiation with a radiocolloid. Br J Heamatol 33:119–127, 1976.
13. Zanesco L: Personal communication.
14. D'Angio GJ, French LA, Stadlan EM, Kieffer SA: Intrathecal radioisotopes for the treatment of brain tumors. Clinical Neurosurgery 15:288–300, 1968.
15. D'Angio GJ: Unpublished observations.

15. Treatment of Meningeal Leukemia: Investigation of New Approaches with Conventional Agents

R. RICCARDI and D.G. POPLACK

Introduction

Treatment of the patient with meningeal leukemia poses a major problem for the pediatric oncologist. Although CNS remission can be achieved in-the majority of cases, remission durations are usually short and most patients suffer subsequent relapse. A major barrier to the identification of successful chemotherapeutic approaches to the treatment of overt meningeal leukemia is the fact that only a few antineoplastic agents are appropriate for intrathecal administration. Although it is well recognized that there is a great need for newer and more effective chemotherapy for CNS leukemia, in the past 20 years no new effective intrathecal chemotherapy agents have been identified. Under this circumstance, one approach to improving CNS treatment is to explore the possibility of utilizing alternative approaches with currently available chemotherapy. In this report we will discuss studies which we have undertaken with two currently available chemotherapeutic agents, cytosine arabinoside and L-asparaginase, in an attempt to define new approaches to the treatment of CNS leukemia.

These experiments were performed in a subhuman primate model developed at the NCI (1). In this model system, a subcutaneously implanted Ommaya reservoir placed over the posterior occiput in the Rhesus monkey is attached to a silicone Pudenz catheter, the tip of which is situated in the fourt ventricle. This system permits sterile ventricular CSF sampling over extended period of time without requiring chronic immobilization, and provides mixing of injected drugs with ventricular CSF (2).

Cytosine arabinoside and tetrahydrouridine

Cytosine arabinoside (Ara-C) is one of the most common antineoplastic agents used to treat CNS leukemia (3). The catabolism of Ara-C is shown in Figure 1. Under ordinary circumstances, the majority of systemically administered Ara-C is rapidly inactivated by cytidine deaminase to the non-toxic compound, uracil arabinoside (Ara-U) (4). Only a small portion of the drug is phosphorylated by deoxycytidine kinase to form, through other sequential conversions, Ara-C

R. Mastrangelo, D.G. Poplack, R. Riccardi (eds), Central Nervous System Leukemia. ISBN 978-94-009-6710-6.
© *1983 Martinus Nijhoff Publishers, Boston.*

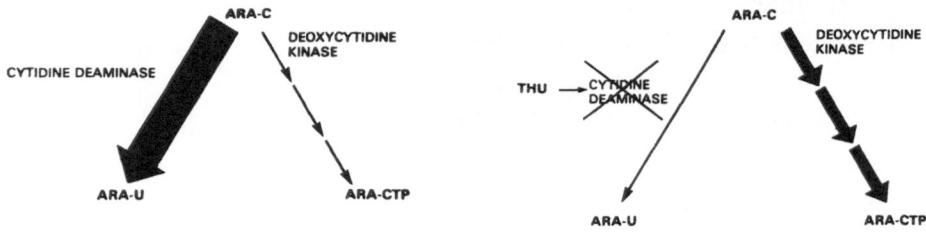

Figure 1 (A). Primary metabolic pathway of cytosine-arabinoside (Ara-C).
Figure 1 (B). Presumed mechanism of tetrahydrouridine (THU) on Ara-C metabolism (See text for details)

triphosphate (Ara-CTP). Ara-CTP is the active metabolite responsible for the inhibition of DNA synthesis. Recent studies have shown that the compound tetrahydrouridine (THU) potentiates the activity of Ara-C, by inhibiting the deamination of Ara-C to Ara-U (5–9). THU also has been demonstrated to increase the net amount of Ara-CTP in cells which have high levels of cytidine deaminase activity (10, 11). The mechanism of action of THU on the catabolism of Ara-C is shown in Figure 1. THU inhibits cytidine deaminase, resulting in a decrease of Ara-U formation and an increase of Ara-CTP. Increases in intracellular Ara-CTP have been correlated with increased cytotoxicity (12–14).

Using the subhuman primate model, we studied the potential of THU to enhance the activity of Ara-C by altering its catabolism following intrathecal administration. These experiments were performed utilizing radiolabeled Ara-C. Levels of Ara-C and its metabolites were measured using thin layer chromatography as previously described (7). In initial experiments, we demonstrated that intrathecal THU in a dose of 6 mg/kg could be administered safely without acute or delayed neurotoxicity. In these experiments, we first studied the pharmacokinetics of Ara-C following intrathecal administration in two monkeys. Following a dose of 1 mg/kg of Ara-C administered via the Ommaya reservoir, serial CSF and blood samples were obtained at periodic time intervals.

As shown in Figure 2, CSF levels of intact Ara-C declined over the first 6 hours with an α half-life of approximately 22 minutes. The α half-life was followed by a β half-life of approximately 116 minutes. Alpha and β half-lives of 32 and 115 minutes respectively were noted when the experiment was repeated in the second animal. The amount of Ara-U present in the CSF increased rapidly following intrathecal Ara-C administration; by 2 hours Ara-C accounted for only 10% of the total radioactivity present in the CSF. Figure 2 also shows the results of the experiments in which we administered intrathecal Ara-C to monkeys who had been pre-treated with intravenous tetrahydrouridine (100 mg/kg). THU pre-treatment resulted in higher levels of Ara-C as a consequence of the inhibitory effect of THU on the catabolism of Ara-C. In this situation, Ara-U formation was markedly decreased and never exceeded 20% of the total radioactivity. We next examined the effect of concomitant intrathecal THU administration upon Ara-C pharmacokinetics in the CSF. As shown in Figure 2, concomitant intrathecal THU administration dramatically altered the CSF pharmacokinetics of Ara-C resulting in a marked alteration in the Ara-C disappearance curve from CSF. Under these experimental conditions, catabolic degradation from Ara-C to Ara-U was virtually completely inhibited. At no time did Ara-U exceed 5% of the total radioactivity. In this situation, intact Ara-C disappeared with a single half-life of approximately 96 minutes in both monkeys.

These studies demonstrate that both IV and IT THU increase the CSF levels of intrathecally administered Ara-C. They also demonstrate that the ability of THU to alter the CSF pharmacokinetics of Ara-C is primarily due to its inhibition of Ara-C deamination. We are presently exploring the possibility of clinically applying this combination in man. At the present time, it is unclear whether THU will have as profound an effect on CSF Ara-C levels in man. However, this approach appears worthy of further study not only because of the ability of THU to alter Ara-C CSF pharmacokinetics, but because of the capacity of THU to increase the concentration of Ara-CTP within malignant cells. This combination

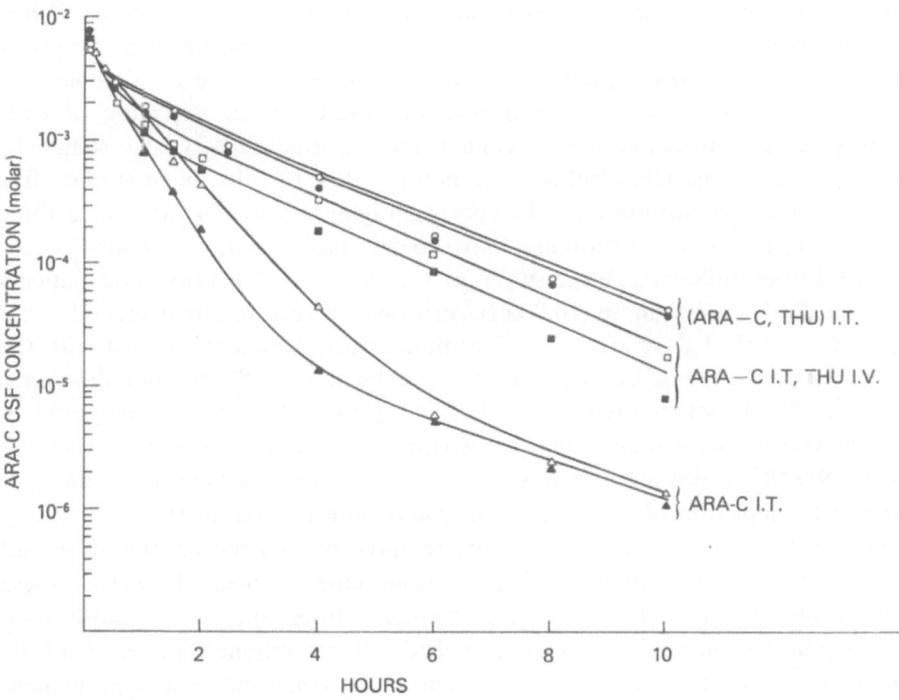

Figure 2. CSF Ara-C concentrations in two monkeys which received IT Ara-C under three different conditions: Ara-C IT alone; Ara-C IT given to monkeys prestreated with IV THU; and Ara-C given simultaneously with THU IT.

may have particular applicability for the treatment of CNS infiltration by malignant cells which possess high levels of cytidine deaminase activity, such as in the case of acute myelongenous leukemia. Further studies are necessary to assess the feasibility and utility of the combination of intrathecal Ara-C and intrathecal THU in man.

L-asparaginase

L-asparaginase is one of the most commonly utilized antineoplastic agents for the treatment of acute lymphoblastic leukemia (15–17). It exerts its antitumor effect by hydrolysis of asparagine selectively effecting leukemic cells which possess low levels of asparagine synthetase. It has been anecdotally reported that patients with CNS leukemia who have received L-asparaginase systemically have obtained CNS remissions (18, 19). Treatment with intrathecal L-asparaginase has also been used successfully in a small number of patients (20). In the present study we investigated the influence of systemically administered L-asparaginase on CSF asparagine levels both in monkeys and in man. In the initial studies we administered L-asparaginase (6000 IU/m^2) IV in monkeys. This dose resulted in plasma asparaginase activity greater than 0.1 IU/ml for at least 24 hours. When these levels of L-asparaginase activity were obtained in plasma, CSF levels of asparagine were totally depleted (see Figure 3). These experiments demonstrate that systemic L-asparaginase administration results in the depletion of CSF asparagine. This mechanism may explain the reported activity of systemic L-asparaginase against CNS leukemia in man (18, 19). In subsequent studies, five patients receiving intramuscular E. coli asparaginase (6000 IU/m^2) on a three times a week schedule, were found to have no detectable asparagine in the CSF for at least a week following the cessation of L-asparaginase therapy. Two patients receiving IV L-asparaginase (10,000 IU/m^2) once a week had undetectable CSF asparagine levels 3 days after the dose. In contrast, 4 patients treated with the same dose and schedule had asparagine detectable in the CSF at 5 to 8 days after the dose. As shown in Figure 3, CSF asparagine both in the monkey and in humans was not detectable if plasma asparaginase activity was greater than 0.1 IU/ml. Results of this study demonstrate that systemic L-asparaginase therapy, through its depletion of CSF asparagine, may be a feasible method of treating meningeal leukemia. Further studies are required to find the optimal dose and schedule to induce depletion of CSF asparagine in man. However, these experiments demonstrate that L-asparaginase doses similar to those used routinely in the clinic are sufficient to deplete CSF asparagine. The results of the present experiments also provide a potential explanation for L-asparaginase related CNS dysfunction (21).

Our work with L-asparaginase, as well as our studies with Ara-C and THU, demonstrate that innovative approaches with currently available conventional

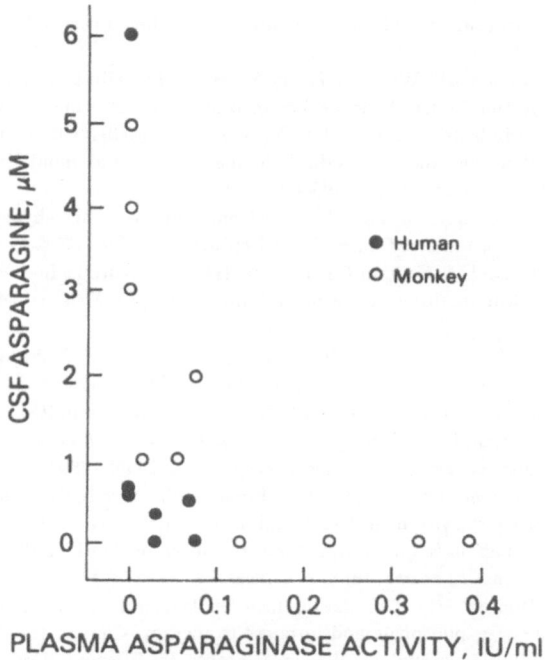

Figure 3. Relationship between plasma asparaginase activity and ventricular CSF asparagine levels. Simultaneous samples obtained from monkeys (O) following IV administration of L-asparaginase (6000 IU/m²) and from patients (●) following L-asparaginase administration at different doses and schedules.

chemotherapeutic agents may increase the therapeutic options available in the treatment of CNS leukemia. However, further clinical studies in man are required before these approaches can be routinely applied.

References

1. Poplack DG, Bleyer WA, Wood JH, Kostolich M, Savitsch JL, Ommaya AK: A primate model for study of methotrexate pharmacokinetics in the central nervous system. Cancer Res 37: 1982–1985, 1977.
2. Wood JH, Poplack DG, Bleyer WA, Ommaya AK: Primate model for the chronic study of intraventricularly or intrathecally administered drugs and intracranial pressure. Science (Wash DC) 195:499–501, 1977.
3. Wang JS, Pratt CB: Intrathecal arabinosylcytosine in meningeal leukemia. Cancer 25:531–536, 1970.
4. Camiener GW, Smith CG: Studies of the enzymatic deamination of cytosine arabinoside. I. Enqyme distribution and species specificity. Biochem Pharmacol 14:1405–1406, 1965.
5. Camiener GW: Studies of the enzymatic deamination of aracytidine. V. Inhibition in vitro and in

vivo by tetrahydrouridine and other reduced pyrimidine nucleosides. Biochem Pharmacol 17:1981–1991, 1968.

6. El Dareer SM, Mellett LB, White V, Tillery K, Mellet LB, Hill DL: Inhibition deamination of ³H-arabinosylcytosine by tetrahydrouridine in BDF₁ mice. Pharmacoligist 16:310, 1974.

7. El Dareer SM, Mulligan LT, Jr, White V, Tillery K, Mellet LB, Hill DL: Distribution of ³H-cytosine arabinoside and its products in mice, dogs, and monkeys and effect of tetrahydrouridine. Cancer Treat Rep 61:395–407, 1977.

8. Kreis W, Hession C, Soricelli A, Scully K: Combinations of tetrahydrouridine and cytosine arabinoside in mouse tumors. Cancer Treat Rep 61:1355–1364, 1977.

9. Kreis W, Woodcock TM, Gordan CS, Krakoff IH: Tetrahydrouridine: Physiologic disposition and effect upon deamination of cytosine arabinoside in man. Cancer Treat Rep 61:1347–1353, 1977.

10. Chou TC, Arlion A, Clarkson BD, Philips FS: Metabolism of 1-β-D-arabinofuranosylcytosine in human leukemic cells. Cancer Res 37:3561–3570, 1977.

11. Ho DHW, Carter JD, Badwin NS, Hester J, McCredie X, Benjamin RS, Freirech EJ, Bodey GP: Effects of tetrahydrouridine on the uptake and metabolism of 1-β-D-arabinofuranosylcytosine in human normal and leukemic cells. Cancer Res 40:2441–2446, 1980.

12. Chou RC, Hutchinson DC, Schmid FA, Phillips FS: Metabolism and selective effects of 1-β-D-arabinofuranosylcytosine in L1210 and host tissues in vivo. Cancer res 35:225–236, 1975.

13. Rustum YM: Metabolism and intracellular retention of 1-β-D-arabinofuranosylcytosine as predictors of response of animal tumors. Cancer Res 38: 543–549, 1978.

14. Rustum WM, Preisler HD: Correlation between leukemic cell retention of 1-β-D-arabinofuranosylcytosine 5'-triphosphate and response to therapy. Cancer Res 39:42–49, 1979.

15. Ertel J, Nesit ME, Hammond D, Weiner J, Sather H: Effective dose of L-asparaginase for induction of remission in previously treted children with acute lymphocytic leukemia: A report from Childrens Cancer Study Group. Cancer Res 39:3893–3896, 1979.

16. Jones B, Holland JF, Glidewell O, Jacquillat C et al: Optimal use of L-asparaginase (NSC-109229) in acute lymphocytic leukemia. Med Pediatr Oncol 3:387–400, 1977.

17. Ortega JA, Nesbit ME, Jr, Donaldson MH, Hittle RE, Weiner J, Karen M, Hammond D: L-Asparaginase, vincristine, and prednisone for induction of first remission in acute lymphocytic leukemia. Cancer Res 37:535–540, 1977.

18. Hill JM, Loeb E, MacLellan A, Khan A, Roberts J, Shields WF, Hill ND: Response to highly purified L-asparaginase during therapy of acute leukemia. Cancer Res 29:1574–1580, 1969.

19. Tallal L, Tan C, Oettgen H, Wallner N, McCarthy M, Helson L, Burchenal J, Karnofsky D, Murphy ML: E. Coli L-asparaginase in the treatment of leukemia and solid tumors in 131 children. Cancer (Phila.) 25:306–310, 1970.

20. Tan C, Oettgen H: Clinical experience with L-asparaginase administered intrathecally. Proc Am Assoc Cancer Res 10:92, 1969.

21. Holland JCB, Fasanell SJ, Ohnuma T: Psychiatric symptoms associated with L-asparaginase administration. J Psychiat Res 10:105–113, 1974.

Subject Index

Ara-U, 132
Arachnoid, 2, 4, 6, 8
Arachnoiditis, 46
Average-risk patients, 28

Bender Visual Motor Gestalt test, 106, 107
Blood-brain-barrier, 2
Bone marrow transplantation, 119
Brain atrophy, 46

C x T, 119
C x T regimen, 120
CCG-101, 11, 36, 124
CCG-141, 27, 34
CCG-141A, 27, 28, 34
CCG-143, 12
CCG-160, 27, 28
CCG-161P, 36
CCSG prognostic groups, 47
CCSG randomized trials, 35
CCSG study, 118
Cerebrospinal fluid (CSF), 2
Children's Cancer Study Group (CCSG),
    11
CNS leukaemia, treatment of overt, 113
CNS prophylaxis
    adverse sequelae of, 95, 105
    alternative methods of, 19
    late consequences of, 19
    neuropsychological functioning of
        children after, 18
CNS relapse, 114, 116, 118
    concurrent, 28
    in boys and girls, 47
    influence of initial white count on the
        incidence of, 44
    isolated, 28
    treatment of isolated, 113
CNS remission duration, 114
CNS sanctuary theory, 39
CNS toxicity
    long-term, 46

observed with IMFRA, 46
Comprehensive psychological assessment,
    84
Correlation between CT brain scans, EEG
    and neuropsychological studies, 109
Cortisol, 86, 99
Cranial irradiation, 114
Cranial nerve palsies, 6
Craniospinal irradiation, 11, 113, 114
CSF, 2, 113
CSF asparagine, 134
CSF cytology, 4
CSF levels of intact Ara-C, 132
CT abnormalities
    decreased attenuation coefficient, 51, 96
    intracerebral calcifications, 51, 96
    ventricular dilatation, 51, 96
CT brain scans, 20, 46, 96, 105, 107
    abnormalities, 21, 96
    structural abnormalities, 88
CT findings, 50, 51
Cytosine arabinoside (Ara-C), 126, 131

EEG, 105, 108
Electroencephalographic assessment, 22
Endocrine evaluation, 85
External beam irradiation, 126
External beam radiation therapy, 11

FSH, 99

Gonadotrophins and gonadal steroids, 87
Growth hormone, 85, 99

High dose methotrexate (HDM), 63
High-risk patients, 28
Histopathologic characteristics, 76
Hydrocephalus, 6, 8
Hypoperfusion, 8
Hypoperfusion encephalopathy, 6
Hypothalamic-pituitary axis, integrity of,
    83

Hypothalamic-pituitary function, 84
    studies, 99

IDM/HDM, 67, 68
IDM, 69
IMFRA, 44, 47
IMFRA CNS prophylaxis schema, 40
IMFRA regimen, 39
Increased risk (IR), 65
Intellectual function, 84, 98
Intellectual performance, 83, 106
Intermediate dose methotrexate (IDM), 63,
    69
Intermittent cranio-spinal irradiation, 14
Intralumbar methotrexate (MTX), 126
Intrathecal radiocolloids, 15
Intraventricular MTX, 126
IQ, 98
    full scale, 98
    performance, 84
    performance scale, 98
    verbal, 84
    verbal scale, 98
IQ scores, 18
IT MTX, 116

Kilovoltage, 12

L-asparaginase, 131, 134
Learning disabilities, 21, 46
Leptomeninges, 2
Leukoencephalopathy, 18, 105
    relationship of radiation and chemotherapy
        to the development, 73
LH, 99
Low dose irradiation, 40
Low risk patients, 28
Lumbar and ventricular CSF concentrations
    of MTX, 119
Lumbar puncture, 123

M-IMFRA, 51
M-IMFRA protocol-treatment schema, 50
Maintenance IT MTX, 30
Medical Research Council, 53
Megavoltage, 12
Memorial Sloan Kettering group, 120
Meningeal leukemia, treatment, new
    approaches, 131
Methotrexate, 113
Mineralizing angiopathy, 46
Mineralizing microangiopathy, 71, 74, 105
    clinical findings, 75
    diagnosis of, 74
    histopathology of, 74

variables associated with the development
    of, 75
Mineralizing vasculopathy, 18
MRC, 113, 116
    first trial, 118
    second trial, 118, 124
    third trial, 118
Myelin basic protein, 22

Neurological abnormalities, 98
Neurological complications of current
    treatment methods, 71
Neuropsychological evaluation, 20
Neuropsychological tests study, 108

Obstruction of CSF flow, 6
Ommaya device, 123
Ommaya reservoir, 116

Pharmaco-kinetically derived intrathecal-
Phosphorous (RP), 15
Pia mater, 2
Pial-glial membrane, 4, 6, 8
    destruction of, 6
Psychometric tests, 105

Radiation therapy methods, 11
Radiation therapy, single courses of, 124
Radio-active colloids, 129
    intraventricular instillation of, 123
Radio-active gold (RG), 15
Results
    of IDM treatment, 66
    of IMFRA treatment, 42
    of M-IMFRA treatment, 50

Seizure, 46
Seizure disorders, 22
St. Jude Children's Research Hospital, 17
St. Jude group, 116
    Standard risk (SR), 65
Structural abnormalities in the brain, 83
Subacute leukoencephalopathy, 71
    clinical features, 72
    histopathologic characteristics, 72
Subacute necrotizing leukomyelopathy, 71,
    76
    etiology of, 79
    histopathologic characteristics, 76
    relationship of clinical and pathological
        features, 77

Tetrahydrouridine, 131
THU, 134
Thyroid function, 86

Total body irradiation, 119
TSH, 99
T_3, 99

UKALL I, 53, 54, 56, 59, 60
UKALL I-V, 54, 55, 58
    trials, 53
UKALL II, 53, 56, 57, 60
UKALL IV, 53
UKALL V, 53, 60
Uracil arabinoside (Ara-U), 131

Ventriculo-lumbar cerebrospinal perfusion,
    119

Wechsler Intelligence Scale for Children
    (WISC), 84, 106
Wechsler intelligence tests and the Bender-
    Gestalt tests of perceptual motor function,
    98
WISC or WRAT, 20